Adaptive Solutions to Personality Disorders

This book explores nidotherapy: the systematic process of changing the physical, social, and personal environment for clients who have failed to respond fully to conventional treatments.

Peter Tyrer argues that clients with personality disorders can improve enormously when placed in the right environment and introduces the process of nidotherapy. The chapters explore methods of matching the patient to the environment, modification of the environment, and patient adaptation, along with case examples and a glossary of key terms. Additionally, the use of ICD-11 classification to understand all aspects of a person's personality is explored to assess personality difficulty, social prescribing, and treatments for severe personality disorder.

This book is essential for psychiatrists, clinical psychologists, and mental health professionals who treat personality disorders, as well as graduate students in clinical psychology courses.

Peter Tyrer is Emeritus Professor of Community Psychiatry in the Division of Psychiatry in the Department of Brain Sciences, Imperial College, London. His extensive body of work includes over 600 original articles and books, primarily focused on subjects such as anxiety, depression, personality disorders, and their respective treatments. In 1990, he developed nidotherapy, an approach involving collaborative and systematic assessment and manipulation of the environment to assist individuals with chronic mental illnesses.

"This passionate and beautifully written book from a leader in community psychiatry makes the case for providing better care for a sadly neglected population. Patients with personality disorders may recover, but those who do not tend to fall within the cracks of the mental health system. Their access to care may be limited by having a difficult personality. Yet, as Tyrer shows, there are evidence-based ways to manage that obstacle. The concept behind nidotherapy is to intervene in ways that better match patients' environment to their personality profile. This concept is well illustrated here by a number of telling case histories. This book will be of great value for mental health clinicians who treat these often-forgotten patients."

Joel Paris, Emeritus Professor of Psychiatry, McGill University. Author of *Social Factors in the Personality Disorders: Finding a Niche*

"In this well written and accessible book, Peter Tyrer captures what might be the essence of personality and its disorders. Synthesising a great breadth of research and his own vast experience combined with research and practice in this field, Tyrer asserts that personality is something we all have, and that, to varying degrees, we are all disordered; but the environment in which we find ourselves will in large part determine the extent to which our disordered personality will cause us harm or, indeed, work in our favour. As Donald Trump has just entered the White House for the second time, and using some illustrative case histories, this sensitively written book makes sense of how environments are so important to anyone with a disordered personality. Rather than turning to therapies such as mentalisation or dialectical behaviour therapies, Tyrer argues, we need to adjust environments for our numerous patients who are largely ignored by the rest of health and mental health to theirs and our detriments. This is a genuinely radical approach which has enormous implications for patients, for psychiatrists for policy makers and for the future of mental health. Read it!"

Tim Kendall, Professor, CBE FRCPsych

"This is a very important book. It opens up a unique perspective on the approach to helping people who have a diagnosis of personality disorder, a concept within itself is open to challenge. Peter Tyrer has been at the forefront on innovative practice in the care and treatment of people with psychological challenges for over 50 years and this book is a must read for all members of the multi-disciplinary team. The link with environment and psychological wellbeing is so often overlooked. Far too often a biological approach is taken to the care and treatment for people with severe and enduring mental illness and in the case of people who are diagnosed with personality disorder they are far too often written off as untreatable.

This book invites the reader to reappraise their thinking in relation to the environment and psychological difficulties and to realise the benefits of Peter Tyrer's approach that, if adopted, will do much to improve the outcomes and offer solutions to some of the challenges that mental health services face."

Dr Peter Carter, former Chief Executive, Royal College of Nursing

Adaptive Solutions to Personality Disorders

Treating Patients with Nidotherapy

Peter Tyrer

Routledge
Taylor & Francis Group

NEW YORK AND LONDON

Designed cover image: Getty Images

First published 2026
by Routledge
605 Third Avenue, New York, NY 10158

and by Routledge
4 Park Square, Milton Park, Abingdon, Oxon, OX14 4RN

Routledge is an imprint of the Taylor & Francis Group, an informa business

ISBN: 9781032909431 (hbk)
ISBN: 9781032869513 (pbk)
ISBN: 9781003560630 (ebk)

DOI: 10.4324/9781003560630

Typeset in Sabon
by Apex CoVantage, LLC

Dedicated to
Ben and Helen
For embracing nidotherapy and seeing it through

Contents

Acknowledgements

This book covers a 60-year period of professional practice in the field of personality and has been helped enormously by many along the way. My thanks are due in my early years to Mike Rutter, who first showed me the importance of personality in childhood development; to Kenneth Rawnsley, who was on the appointments committee of my first senior post and encouraged me to follow my nose; and James Gibbons for reinforcing this advice later. More recently, I would like to thank all my colleagues on our ICD-11 working group for the revision of personality disorders, especially Mike Crawford, Lee Anna Clark, Alireza Farnam, Andrea Fossati, Dusica Lecic-Tosevski, and Roger Mulder, and to Geoff Reed for expert diplomatic guidance. Joel Paris in Montreal has contributed greatly to the literature on personality disorder and he has helped greatly in getting a full understanding of the borderline concept in Chapter 4. Finally, and more recently still, I have valued greatly the support given to all at our charity, NIDUS-UK, by Carl and Rin on their rehabilitation barge at Isleworth (http://www.cathja.org), Dr Catherine Gardiner in her GP practice in Rochester, Dr Peter Carter for not being afraid to take on the battle for reform for the NHS, our other NIDUS-UK trustees for not giving up on me, and Professor Tim Kendall for his efforts to support change at the top (as well as giving me details of improved Sheffield architecture). A final thanks to Glenn Roberts for allowing me to stir the memory of Anthea in Chapter 16 and to use part of the text I have sent him. It was Anthea who, with a little help from Phil Harrison-Read, helped me understand the fundamental message of nidotherapy, which Stefano Pallanti (2010) has summarised so well as 'the ultimate personalized medicine, because its primary therapeutic strategy is the full appreciation of the patient as a unique person in his or her own environment'.

Reference

Pallanti S (2010). *American Journal of Psychiatry*, 167, 871. Nidotherapy: Harmonising the environment with the patient.

Introduction

The title of this book may puzzle. Most people have a view about personality and personality disorder that can be expressed, rather baldly, as 'personality describes us as we are and does not change much, and as personality disorder is similar but creates problems it does not change much either'. Therefore, we should always regard personality disorder as permanent and hope that nobody ever regards us as personality disordered, as it appears to be a life sentence.

This is quite wrong, and the task of this book is to put it right. It is quite an undertaking. I have three aims: to remove the stigma attached to disordered personalities, to show their oft-hidden strengths and advantages, and to describe how a form of environmental management, nidotherapy, can help them be free of disorder.

My two robust assistants in this endeavour are the new classification of personality dysfunction, the 11th International Classification of Disease (ICD-11) (World Health Organisation, 2024) and the principles of adaptation. The first of these achieves the elimination of stigma. What a bold claim, you say; it cannot possibly be true. But stigma only applies when it allows one group of people to be separated from another—the original stigma was a mark by a pointed instrument that was used as identification—and, when this is removed, stigma disappears. The ICD-11 classification, discussed in great detail later, is not just a dry document listing minor changes. It is based on scientific data showing most people in the world have some degree of personality dysfunction (Yang et al., 2010; Bach et al., 2023).

King Edward VII created ripples in 1902 when he repeated the mantra 'we are all socialists now'. King Charles III could do the same by saying 'we are all personality disordered now', and, given his support for causes that start eccentric and then become mainstream, he may well utter this at some point. The evidence from epidemiology, a part of science that merely records and is unbiased, shows that only a small minority of the population have no personality difficulties. This does not mean we are a dysfunctional people; it just means we can all have problems in dealing with others, and these can cause distress. Once we accept this as part of personality, stigma will fade away.

The advantages of personality disorder are not immediately apparent. But when you look behind the unflattering descriptions of personality problems there is hidden merit. Here, for example, are descriptions of some of the personality characteristics, commonly called traits, that constitute an assessment called SPAN-DOC, short for Structured Personality Assessment from Notes and Documents (Tyrer & Clark, 2007).

Trait 3: Anger/irritability

This trait, when expressed prominently, is summarised as 'angry and argumentative attitudes towards others; poor ability to compromise or come to terms with views that are not entirely consonant with one's own; angers easily and has difficulty controlling his/her temper once aroused; frequently gets into verbal conflicts; holds a grudge after conflicts occur'.

Trait 6: Suspiciousness/mistrust

'Consistently mistrustful and doubtful of others' intentions; hides feelings from others, does not let others get to know him/her well, suspicious of being taken advantage of; believes that people often lie to and/or try to make him/her look foolish or bad'.

Trait 7: Hypersensitivity

'Persistent excessive touchiness and sensitivity to (perceived) criticism; frequently takes offence against apparent slights; easily aggravated; prickly; consequently is often disappointed in, or feels betrayed by, others'.

Trait 8: Aggression

'Persistent, easily generated unprovoked physical aggression towards properties or individuals; enjoys others' aggression and physical fights; enjoys engendering fear in others'.

Trait 15: Entitlement

'Believes self to be special and that others should envy him/her; sees him/herself as consistently "in the right"; at higher levels, feels self more deserving than others and entitled to whatever he/she wants; expects all requests to be granted'.

Trait 16: Exhibitionism

'Attention-seeking: desires/expects to be the centre of attention; acts and dresses to gain and maintain others' attention; at higher levels, frequently engages in public behaviours designed to attract attention (e.g., overt flirting, speaking/performing in public)'.

Trait 20: Sensation/novelty seeking

'Constant need for new and greater stimulation; continual seeking of increased sensation and novelty; enjoys taking risks and engaging in dangerous activities; at higher levels, sensation seeking overrides even basic safety measures'.

Trait 21: Impulsivity

'Acts without thought for consequences; does and says the first thing that comes to mind without considering potential behavioural outcomes, negative consequences, or effects on others; at lower levels may appear spontaneous and carefree; whereas those at higher levels appear reckless and disorganised'.

Trait 23: Callousness

'Indifference and insensitivity to needs of others; exploits and revels in others' suffering. indifferent to others, 'little empathy, doesn't seem to care about other people, laughs at others' misfortune'.

Trait 24: Irresponsibility

'Failure to honour obligations and duties, including lack of punctuality and poor quality performance; thoughtless, even reckless, disregard for the needs, wishes, and safety of others and own safety, may show passive-aggressive behaviour to evade responsibilities and when more serious is overtly deceitful and manipulative'.

Each of these is portrayed in a negative light. But if you look at the evolution of mankind, you can find times when these features have been advantageous for survival and protection, and even now, there are some in positions of authority who can use these traits to advantage. One does not have to look very far; Donald Trump comes to mind. Looking back, Neanderthal man, protecting his family and living in a cave, needed to be able to show anger and be aggressive when threatened, to be suspicious of the intentions of others, and to have especial sensitivity to threat. The more dominant members of the tribe needed to be self-important and expect fealty from others so their numbers could increase. If their tribe needed more space to grow, this could involve the elimination of others by deception, manipulation, and planned aggression. Genghis Khan did not conquer vast areas of Asia by being upright, proper, and gentle; he was ruthless, aggressive, determined, and sometimes quite nasty. All the traits listed here were advantageous at his time in history.

Environments in the past were very different from those at present, but our personalities have not yet learnt to adapt, and we still maintain some of our Neanderthal attitudes in a world that has moved on. When these dominate our daily function, they lead to distress and dysfunction, both to the person concerned and to others. This is because there is a mismatch; long-standing primitive characteristics are no longer appropriate in today's world.

This is the point at which adaptive solutions are needed. These can be provided by nidotherapy, which allows all aspects of the environment to be reassessed and, where necessary, changed to make a better fit for the person. We practise nidotherapy in our own lives, and, when we do, we need not give it a fancy title. We decide to move into occupations that best fit our talents, move to places where we feel secure and comfortable, and find friends who are mutually reinforcing and satisfying. But those with personality problems do not get this positive reinforcement. They do not fit in, they are multi-shaped pegs in ill-fitting holes, and as a consequence they and others suffer. Finding successful adaptive strategies for them is difficult, and this is why this book has been written. Extra help is needed to examine all aspects of the environment—place, people, and person—to try and find a better match for the personality. Once a better match is identified, former negative personality features become positive. This is followed by greater self-confidence and self-esteem, and, what is most important, personality becomes an asset rather than a problem. You will read example after example of this in this book. The changes in nidotherapy are decided by the person concerned; they are not forced in from outside, and so they always remain under personal control.

This book examines adaptive solutions for all personality disorders, not just a select few. When we look at the official textbook descriptions of treatments for personality disorder, we try to be optimistic, but we are really in a desert of despond. Only a few very intensive treatments exist for a small proportion of people collectively described as borderline, a word that creates only chaos and confusion, and for the rest, we only offer a morsel or two to justify our efforts. Quite simply, if there were many widely used treatments for personality disorder that were clearly effective. there would be no need for this book. But there are not. I do not want to criticise the major treatments that do exist as a great deal of effort has gone into developing and improving them. They are doubtlessly of some value but *there are too many people wanting them and the intensity of the treatments is such that the demand will never be satisfied* (Duggan & Tyrer, 2022). Adaptive solutions are described in this book for all parts of personality dysfunction, for those who are isolated and detached, those who are angry and frustrated, those who labour under the weight of anxiety and doubt, and those who rush in where angels fear to tread. These solutions can be carried out individually or with the help of others; in nidotherapy practice, external help is often needed.

There are other approaches that adopt the strategy of environmental change. One of these is social prescribing, an unfortunately named intervention as it implies a medical top-down intervention similar to a drug prescription. But it is very different from this. Those referred to this service see a link worker who offers advice about environmental options available in the local community, and the link worker is usually well versed in those that might be available. Most of those referred have been attending medical and mental health services frequently and have made little or no improvement, so everyone has become frustrated.

But social prescribing has a very broad brush and is not in any way focused on helping those with personality problems, even though at times their interventions happen to be adaptive and provide a custom-made solution. But social prescribing has no scientific base and is very poorly researched, and because the presentations cover a complete range of problems from trivial worries to intractable personality difficulties, social prescribers are often left in a quandary and have little in the way of help available from others. There is also a worry that those who might be most helped are never referred. As two very active supporters of social psychiatry put it,

> Social prescribing is poorly defined and there is little evidence for its effectiveness. It cannot address the social determinants of mental health and it is unlikely to produce enduring change for that part of the population that suffers the worst physical and mental health, namely the most deprived and marginalised. It has emerged at a time of growing health inequity.
>
> (Poole & Huxley, 2024)

But social prescribing represents a start and needs support and encouragement. I suggest that nidotherapy can be formulated as a more sophisticated form of social prescribing (Tyrer, 2019) that is of particular value for those with personality problems.

The message from this book is optimistic. here we have a simple form of management that has been shown to be cost effective—it delivers much and costs very little and so is approved by health economists (Ranger et al., 2009; Tyrer et al., 2011; Barrett & Tyrer, 2012); the alternative options are much more expensive (Barrett et al., 2009). Although personality problems are very common and sometimes create much difficulty, we can make a difference with nidotherapy. Adaptation can be taught; it is not labour intensive and does not need large programmes of training, and significant elements of it are common sense. Adaptation to the environment is the core of nidotherapy, and it needs emphasising that it can be carried out by everyone, irrespective of their education or training, as successful nidotherapy comes from the person inside, not the expert in the wings. People with personality problems, their relatives and friends, and their colleagues in other walks of life, can all practise nidotherapy in different ways, and when all work together in unison, it is highly successful.

But that is enough promotion. The rest of this book shows the power of adaptive solutions by example. Sceptics are common when advances in the treatment of personality disorder are claimed. I am a great supporter of scepticism as it is the enemy of dogma, but after reading about the power of adaptation, I trust scepticism will melt away.

Peter Tyrer
March 2025

References

Bach B, Simonsen E, Kongerslev MT, Bo S, Hastrup LH, Simonsen S, et al. (2023). ICD-11 personality disorder features in the Danish general population: cut-offs and prevalence rates for severity levels. *Psychiatry Research*, 328, 115484.

Barrett B, Byford S, Seivewright H, Cooper S, Duggan C & Tyrer P (2009). The assessment of dangerous and severe personality disorder: service use, cost and consequences. *Forensic Psychology and Psychiatry*, 20, 120–131.

Barrett B & Tyrer P (2012). The cost-effectiveness of the Dangerous and Severe Personality Disorder Programme. *Criminal Behaviour & Mental Health*, 22, 202–209.

Duggan C & Tyrer P (2022). Specialist teams as constituted are unsatisfactory for treating people with personality disorders. *BJPsych Bulletin*, 46, 100–102.

Poole R & Huxley P (2024). Social prescribing: an inadequate response to the degradation of social care in mental health. *BJPsych Bulletin*, 48, 30–33.

Ranger M, Tyrer P, Miloseska K, Fourie H, Khaleel I, North B, et al. (2009). Cost-effectiveness of nidotherapy for comorbid personality disorder and severe mental illness: randomized controlled trial. *Epidemiologia e Psichiatria Sociale*, 18, 128–136.

Tyrer P (2019). Nidotherapy: a cost-effective systematic environmental treatment. *World Psychiatry*, 18, 144–145.

Tyrer P & Clark L-A (2007). *Schedule for Personality Assessment from Notes and Documents (SPAN-DOC)*. Imperial College, London & University of Notre Dame, Indiana.

Tyrer P, Miloševska K, Whittington C, Ranger M, Khaleel I, Crawford M, et al. (2011). Nidotherapy in the treatment of substance misuse, psychosis and personality disorder: secondary analysis of a controlled trial. *The Psychiatrist*, 35, 9–14.

World Health Organisation (2024). *Clinical Descriptions and Diagnostic Requirements for ICD-11 Mental, Behavioural and Neurodevelopmental Disorders*. WHO: Geneva.

Yang M, Coid J & Tyrer P (2010). A national survey of personality pathology recorded by severity. *British Journal of Psychiatry*, 197, 193–199.

Chapter 1

Defining current thinking in personality disorders and nidotherapy

Two complex subjects, personality disorders and nidotherapy, are introduced in this chapter. These terms must be treated with a modicum of caution. The diagnosis of personality disorder is too often regarded as a diagnosis of rejection rather than one of promise. It is not a happy word couplet. People love 'personality' as it describes the essence of a person, but when you add 'disorder', it becomes offensive. In a flash, the prince of personality is transformed into a toad of disorder once the two are combined. But we have to live with language, and there is no point in trying to change words when we all understand the essence of the subject. Ask any person who treats people with intellectual disability whether changing the names of this group of people from idiot to moron to mental subnormality and handicap, to learning disability and intellectual disability, and finally to the ultimate suppressor of offence, a bowdlerised acronym such as PWID (people with intellectual disability) has changed attitudes, and they will answer 'none'. Attitudes have changed, but the changes occurred first, the new names followed, and attitudes often remained. In this book, personality disorder is being re-erected as a positive term that gives hope and encouragement, but it will not be an easy task to convince many that it is not just a term of stigma, as opinions are so entrenched. Please give personality disorder a fair chance by reading carefully and then spreading the optimistic word.

Nidotherapy does not have the same stigma as personality disorder as it is a new term that is not well known. It was originally defined as 'a collaborative treatment involving the systematic assessment and modification of the environment to minimise the impact of any form of mental disorder on the individual or on society' (Tyrer et al., 2003). This definition remains largely true, but the word 'treatment' is better changed to 'approach' as nidotherapy is not a treatment in the formal sense as everybody can have access to it. Whenever we change our jobs, our accommodation, our partners and friends, and our lives for the better we are practising nidotherapy.

DOI: 10.4324/9781003560630-1

But when we become stuck in our personal, social, and physical environments and become unwell or frustrated, a more formal variety of nidotherapy is needed. This can come from self-examination, help from friends and relatives, or help from professionals. It is with the last group that nidotherapy comes into its own as a useful guide. There are full accounts of nidotherapy published elsewhere, including books (Akerman et al., 2018; Tyrer, 2009, 2018; Tyrer & Tyrer, 2018), clinical trials (Ranger et al., 2009; Tyrer et al., 2017), qualitative studies (Spencer et al., 2010; Ahmed & Tyrer, 2024), and case reports (Spears et al., 2017; Tyrer & Bajaj, 2005), and in Chapter 7, I explain its aims in detail.

But at this point, there needs to be a short explanation of why nidotherapy is particularly suited to the management of personality disorder. It is because all personality problems constitute interactions between a person and the environment, which covers place, people, and self. When we come across people with personality disorder, we see a mismatch between person and environment. It is a mismatch that has to involve other people; a person with mental illness still has the illness wherever he or she is placed, but someone with personality disorder needs someone else for the disorder to be manifest. So when totally alone in the world, all those with personality disorder lose their diagnosis; other diagnoses stay the same.

The perceived universal negative interaction with others that creates the diagnosis is the essential part of the personality problem, and, unlike simple nidotherapy—wanting a change and creating the circumstances to implement it—the person troubled with the personality problem does not have a quick and easy answer. Part of this is central to the nature of personality dysfunction, the distorted self-awareness that prevents people from seeing why their interactions with others are damaging. It is very easy to blame others when something goes wrong; the person with a personality disorder is prone to this error, feeling that it is others, not him or her, who need to change. But some change in the physical or social environment is recognised to be important, and, in the case of personality disorder, it assumes greater relevance than in other disorders when treatment of symptoms becomes the dominant aim. With personality problems, adaptation is needed; Svrakic et al. (2009) have even suggested that personality disorders should be relabelled adaptation disorders.

Because there is a lot of confusion about the central features of personality disorder, these need to be clarified first. There is a more comprehensive account elsewhere (Tyrer & Mulder, 2022), but some of the essentials need to be repeated. As a start, please try and be open minded about the subject and not to be too swayed by what you have read elsewhere, much of which is dogma and opinion and, quite simply, wrong headed. Personality disorder is not a permanent state, it does not need to ruin your life, it is often associated with valuable strengths, it has assets that those without personality problems lack, and it can be used positively to build an optimistic future.

The essence of personality disorder

I have to start this section by explaining why personality disorder has been reclassified recently and why so many of past terms are now defunct. Classification and diagnosis are often regarded as dull or offensive. They come over as dull when they make statements that are so obvious there seems no point in repeating them—'we knew all this already', patronising; 'that's obvious, tell us something new'; and annoyance: 'Are you really saying I have to change my practice just because a distant committee says so?' Diagnosis is sometimes regarded as an offensive medical label by many who think of it as a means of preventing the shift to understanding the real meaning of people's stories (Boyle & Johnstone, 2020). I am not going to rehash these arguments, only to say that separating people into groups that have common features is a practice that aids communication. Diagnosis is neither right nor wrong; it is merely useful for understanding.

I am going to illustrate why diagnosis or grouping or categorising or listing, whatever you choose to call it, is valuable in the field of personality. I describe five people—Arthur, Bethany, Callum, Dorothea and Eric—who represent the different levels of personality pathology that are included in ICD-11 (the 11th Revision of the International Classification of Diseases), introduced in 2022 and fully documented in 2024 (World Health Organisation, 2024). You will come across them again in later chapters, and you will get to know them well.

Arthur

Arthur is 30. He is a successful junior executive in a large publishing company and is hoping for further promotion. He has had several girl-friends in the last ten years and was hoping to be married by now, but the right person does not seem to have come along. He is personable and reasonably attractive and has had no problems in developing romantic relationships, but in time, they tend to go cold. His friends tell him he is too fussy, but he disputes that—he expects a marriage to last for life, so the decision and choice are highly important.

He is conventional and likes to be one of the crowd. Standing out in any way is not for him; he views it as a form of showing off. He likes watching James Bond films on TV, supports Manchester City but does not go to see games, and has two weeks holiday in Majorca every summer. He is not great at conversations and prefers to listen to others as it is less demanding.

Bethany

Bethany is 28 and works as an assistant in a firm specializing in graphic design. She is about to get married to one of the partners in the firm and is looking forward to a bright future. She dresses neatly and smartly, and her coiffured hair is universally admired as a work of art. She takes the same degree of care in her work as with her appearance but is not particularly liked by her colleagues as they often are criticised and belittled by her when they do not come up to her high standards. When she is away from work, she is a sparkling companion and gets on well with all.

Callum

Callum is 29. He is a professional footballer playing in one of the lower divisions in the Football League. He realises he will never be a top-class player and wants to maximise his earnings before retirement in a few years time. He has developed a relationship with a betting group, and there are suspicions that his performance on the field is linked to bets made by this group, but nothing has been proved. Callum is often extravagant in his relationships with women, feeling he is exceptionally attractive, and likes to show off in front of his many girl-friends. His relationships seldom last long, and he has been accused of violence toward his former fiancée, often after he has been drinking heavily. He accepts that he often acts impulsively and cannot control his temper but blames this on alcohol.

Dorothea

Dorothea is 30. She has always been a mercurial character and never quite knows where she is going in life. She had high ambitions as a teenager, but whenever any of these did not turn out as expected, she over-reacted and felt she was useless and inadequate. At these times, ever since the age of 16, she self-harmed by cutting herself. She did this as a way of relieving tension, and it has now become a habit, but at times she has cut too deeply, has bled profusely, and had to be seen at hospital. She has never married but has had a number of intense relationships that have all ended in acrimony. She blames her 'intense emotions' for these breakdowns but also feels she is attracted to the wrong men. She works in the fashion industry and has had many different jobs, always starting with enthusiasm but ending with disillusion.

Eric

Eric is aged 30 and is currently in prison for assault and battery. He was abandoned as a child and subsequently fostered by three different foster parents, all of whom found him difficult and aggressive and so could not continue to look after him. He played truant repeatedly at school, was expelled from two of them for fighting, and never properly completed his education. Since the age of 18, he has had been convicted of six offences—rape, assault and battery, burglary and armed robbery, and has spent five years in prison in total for these offences. He has had two partners, but both relationships broke down because he was over-possessive and violent.

These five people are very different. Their personalities separate them, as do their life stories. Nobody could claim that their problems can be properly summarised in the two or three words of a diagnosis, but we have to separate them in some way from each other as they are so different. For most of the last 100 years, we have made this separation by putting each person into a category, a simple summary of a personality type. So we can examine our five examples in this way. Arthur seems to be very normal; we cannot categorise him as disordered in any way, although some people may think he is just a little bit boring. Bethany is also well put together, and, although she is a bit of a fusspot who can irritate people because of her high standards, most can live with this without getting upset. Callum is different. He flirts with criminality, is inconsistent in his behaviour, is violent in some of his relationships, and is egotistical. He could readily be classified as a sociopath and labelled with an antisocial or narcissistic personality disorder. Dorothea arouses sympathy. She has good intentions, but everything in her life tends to go wrong, her relationships keep on breaking down, and she has got into the habit of repeatedly harming herself. As her emotional instability predominates, she immediately attracts the diagnosis of borderline personality disorder. Eric is the most abnormal of the five. He had a bad start in life but seems determined to let it continue in the same vein. His repeated offending and violent behaviour now seem to on a recurring path, and it will be hard to shift it. He also can readily be classified as a psychopath, sociopath, or antisocial personality.

But how much do these diagnostic labels help? Not very much. They give the same diagnosis to Callum and Eric, even though they are very different people. The diagnosis of borderline personality disorder is also not very informative. It seems to apply to lots of people and does not tell us much about Dorothea as a person. It also implies there is no difference between Arthur and Bethany, but there is. These labels are also very stigmatic and offensive. If the antisocial and borderline diagnoses were replaced by a sticker saying 'this person is bad news, stay away' it would summarise the reaction they create.

There is a better way of describing personality variation. All the evidence points toward personality problems being best presented as a spectrum from normal personality function at one extreme and severe personality disorder at the other. This model (Tyrer et al., 2011) was criticised as too radical by many when it was first introduced (Bateman, 2011; Davidson, 2011) but has now been generally accepted as a better way of classifying most mental disorders (Kotov et al., 2017). This makes sense as there have been very few disorders in which key differences are found between those with and without different diagnoses. No blood test, no brain scan or investigation, no psychological test, no cognitive task, and no intelligence test is able to distinguish between normal and abnormal personalities. Put another way, all of us have the capacity to act as though we had a personality disorder. Lord David Owen, formerly a psychiatrist at St Thomas's Hospital in London, where we both worked for the same consultant, described the hubris syndrome (Owen, 2008, 2012), the change in personality created by 'the intoxication of power', as an acquired personality disorder. I dislike the impression that such a change is a permanent one, but it does illustrate that when put in certain environments, personalities can change for the worse rather than for the better. The key safeguards against personalities getting out of control are personal reflection and critical feedback from others, but when the very powerful surround themselves with like minds these safeguards melt away. Donald Trump beware; loyal followers are not enough.

The spectrum of personality needs to have defining points to help decide where each individual stands at any one time. The World Health Organisation has classified all illnesses since 1900, and this includes mental disorders. And, please note, if the word 'disorder' offends you, it is just the universal term used to describe any problem, physical or mental, that creates suffering or shortens life. I am trying to use it sparingly throughout this book, but it cannot be ignored.

The first task is to distinguish personality disorder from no personality disorder. If you accept that all personality problems lie on a spectrum, the creation of a dividing line in this way is arbitrary; it has very little meaning.

Nonetheless, we have to create a definition of personality disorder, not least for legal reasons. The law gives special attention to this subject as careful assessment can lead to important differences in sentencing when offences are committed.

This is the latest formal definition of personality disorder as defined by the World Health Organisation in its Clinical Descriptions and Diagnostic Guidelines

---

Box 1.1   The formal definition of personality disorder in ICD-11

World Health Organisation definition

An enduring disturbance characterised by problems in functioning of aspects of the self (e.g. identity, self-worth, accuracy of self-view, self-direction) and/or interpersonal dysfunction (e.g. ability to develop and maintain close and mutually satisfying relationships, ability to understand others' perspectives and to manage conflict in relationships) is required for diagnosis.

- The disturbance has persisted over an extended period of time (e.g. lasting 2 years or more).
- The disturbance is manifested in patterns of cognition, emotional experience, emotional expression and behaviour that are maladaptive (e.g. inflexible or poorly regulated).
- The disturbance is manifested across a range of personal and social situations (i.e. is not limited to specific relationships or social roles), although it may be consistently evoked by particular types of circumstances and not others.
- The symptoms are not due to the direct effects of a medication or substance, including withdrawal effects, and are not better accounted for by another mental disorder, a disease of the nervous system or another medical condition.

The additional requirement is that the disturbance is associated with substantial distress or significant impairment in personal, family, social, educational, occupational, or other important areas of functioning (this also applies to many other disorders) and the caveat that personality disorder should not be diagnosed if the patterns of behaviour characterising the personality disturbance are developmentally appropriate (e.g. problems related to establishing an independent self-identity during adolescence) or can be explained primarily by social or cultural factors, including socio-political conflict (World Health Organisation, 2024, p. 554).

The concepts described here are not easy to define. They are not classical symptoms, even though they are given that label; they are not clear-cut behaviours like obsessional checking; and they also seem to include concepts such as self-identity that are odd and mysterious to the average clinician or person in the street. So when a clinician, a lawyer, a friend or neighbour, or even a family member wants to ascribe, judge, or assess whether a person has a personality problem, each has a big task on their hands.

But how can this be done quickly and efficiently? If you read the schedules of personality assessment such as the International Personality Disorder Examination (IPDE) (Loranger et al., 1994), you will see over 400 questions about personality status. When I was in Luxembourg in 1987 with an international group working our way through each question in the IPDE, we often wondered if this instrument—some called it The Monster—would ever be used. But used it was, widely and for many years, but not by the thousands of clinicians who see people with personality problems every day of their lives. It was an instrument used by specialists in personality disorder and in research studies, but not by GPs or general psychiatrists. It also had an unfortunate ambience. As one of my exasperated Scandinavian colleagues put it during questioning, 'I do not like asking "Are you the son of a bitch?" 450 times'.

But the IPDE was assessing the old personality disorder classifications, which have become outdated labels that are generally considered abusive and generate stigma, but they have been bandied about so widely they have lost their sting (ask Donald Trump). The new revision of the World Health Organisation classification, mentioned earlier, is the eleventh version of the International Classification of Diseases (ICD-11), the first done in 1900. The ICD-11 classification has dispensed with all the old outworn categories and replaced them with a dimensional system, a spectrum of pathology based entirely on severity. The definition provided here is only the central part of the ICD-11 system, but on either side, we have lesser and more severe levels of personality problems that complete the spectrum (Figure 1.1). It also has shorter instruments to record its features (Moran et al., 2003; Oltmann & Widiger, 2018; Olajide et al., 2018; Bach et al., 2021; Kim et al., 2021).

The advantage of a spectrum is that it includes everybody, and each has to have a single position somewhere. The old system of classification had people bouncing from one diagnosis to another like a flashing manic pin-ball machine, sometimes finishing up with five or six different diagnoses. The spectrum does not allow diagnoses to cohabit. It is forced to place anchor points to assist clinicians in deciding which compartment of the spectrum each person should occupy. These are not fixed points, but they are important to identify, and six elements of the personality problem need to be examined closely (Table 1.1).

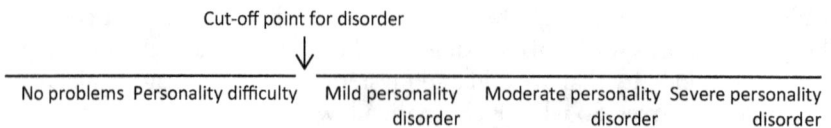

Cut-off point for disorder

| No problems | Personality difficulty | Mild personality disorder | Moderate personality disorder | Severe personality disorder |

Figure 1.1 The ICD-11 classification of personality problems

Table 1.1 Six elements of severity of personality problems

Ability to perform societal roles
Degree of distorted self-perception
Degree of interpersonal social dysfunction
Mental state comorbidity
Risk of harm to self or others
Situational aspects

These six elements can be compared easily by looking at each of them for the five people listed earlier. Arthur does not have problems with any of these—he is personable, performing well in his job, has good relationships with all, is not mentally ill, seems to have no weak spots, and is certainly not at risk of any type of harm. He is almost too nice to be true—J.D. Salinger's Holden Caulfield in *Catcher in the Rye* would no doubt call him a 'goddam phony'—but Holden would be in a minority. Arthur is a popular guy.

Bethany is also well put together in more ways than one. She is neat, well-organised, and efficient, and in most situations, she is a charming companion. But she is ever so slightly bossy, and at work, she creates a mild level of conflict that is clearly linked to her personality. But this has no effect on her other societal roles or her general functioning.

Callum is different. He is a successful footballer, but his life is in danger of going seriously wrong. He is close to criminal behaviour, has a distorted high opinion of himself, is on the road toward alcohol dependence, and has a propensity to be violent. All these elements add to his personality pathology, so he is very different from Bethany.

Dorothea has similar difficulties, but these are more serious as they include harm, and harm of any sort raises the diagnostic stakes as the integrity of the individual or others is at risk, a risk that can include death. So it is not surprising that the problems Dorothea presents make the level of severity higher. It is also relevant that she is clearly suffering more in a way that Callum is not.

Eric is much worse. All six of the elements listed earlier are present—he has no role in society as a repeat felon, he does not seem to have any understanding that his life story is self-destructive, his relationships with others are almost pure conflict, he is disturbed mentally, and he is a serious risk to the health of others as he is so aggressive.

So even the most sceptical of folk who recoil at the word 'diagnosis' would agree with the following conclusion (Figure 1.2).

The big problem every person has when trying to decide where somebody is on this spectrum is the implication of blame. The further away you are from normality, the greater the likelihood you will be thought of

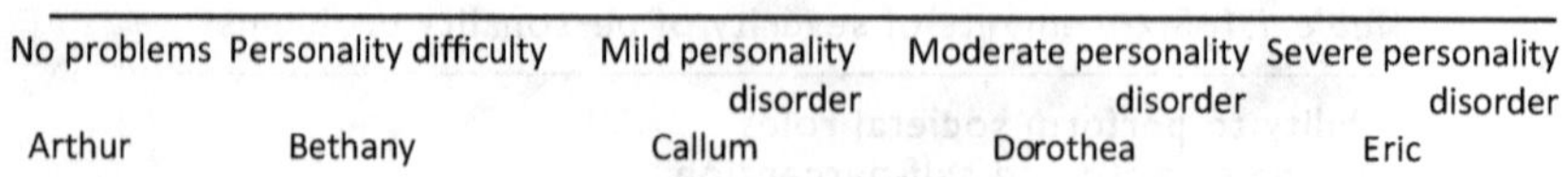

No problems	Personality difficulty	Mild personality disorder	Moderate personality disorder	Severe personality disorder
Arthur	Bethany	Callum	Dorothea	Eric

Figure 1.2 Separation of personalities in ICD-11

as a nasty person whose troubles are all your own fault and may be even be deserved. If you are anxious or depressed, you deserve sympathy and understanding, but if you have a disturbed personality, you are beyond the pale. As Stephen Fry puts it, to be described as having a personality disorder 'threatens our sense of self and the very ownership of who we are' (Fry, 2018).

The consequence of the pernicious implications of personality pathology leads to most people ignoring it, unless you happen to be appearing in court when all restraint seems to be lost. These implications are not lost on the general public. Call me anxious, impulsive, psychotic, angry, autistic, or obsessional if you will, but call me personality disordered at your peril.

So psychiatrists cannot say openly to most people, 'I think you have a personality disorder, and here are my reasons'. The second part of the sentence is lost as it is overtaken by anger. So I have learnt over many years of practice by assessing personality problems in a slightly different way.

I am not saying this is necessarily the best way, but it has kept me out of trouble. This is the approach I use when assessing personality in the patients I meet in practice, and this could be a guide for all who are in a similar position, wanting to be honest and not wishing to offend. You will note I start on positive features; these are almost always present and need to be exposed.

After a personal introduction—always make it personal—you ask:

'Would you like to summarise the sort of person you are, particularly stressing your strengths and any difficulties you have encountered?'

You will get a clue what is going on, but often you get a reply that is not that informative—'I'm pretty ordinary really, just get on with things', and so you have to probe with further questions.

'Do you get on well with other people in your daily life?'

'Are there any people you tend to avoid or are bothered to be in their company?'

'Have difficulties with other people caused any serious problems in your life to date?'

'To what extent do you think they have been caused by others or you yourself?'

'Do you feel you have not been treated fairly by others?'

The answers to these questions may allow you to make a provisional assessment of personality. This can first be grouped into five levels of interpersonal functioning for (a) presence of conflict and (b) personal contribution. The second of these is more difficult to assess. Some people are treated badly and have a right to complain, but often the way in which the person has behaved has been the main source of trouble.

A.   Presence of conflict

1 No evidence of personality conflict from answers
2 Admitted problems but explanations for them suggest most are very minor
3 Some evidence of interpersonal conflict with short-term negative consequences for individual
4 Considerable evidence of interpersonal conflict with long-term negative consequences for individual and others
5 Widespread evidence of interpersonal conflict with impact on all areas of life for both individual and others

B.   Personal contribution

1 No evidence of personality contribution to any of the described difficulties
2 Slight evidence that individual has contributed in minor part to any difficulties
3 Some clear evidence of contribution that individual is responsible, at least in part, for the difficulties described
4 Considerable evidence that the individual is responsible to a large extent for creating interpersonal difficulties
5 Widespread evidence that the individual has be the main reason for the difficulties described
Take the mean score of these two ratings for **interpersonal conflict**.

• ☐ Take mean of presence and personal contribution scores

Although there can be many areas of conflict, they may only take place with one or two people. Obviously, if one of those people is someone you work or mix with very closely, the problem may be a considerable one, but if the difficulties are only with that person, the impact is much less than when the conflict is general. You need to tease out the situations and the people with whom the conflict occurs. If there is only one person with whom you have the conflict, the personality problem may be not your problem at all, but do not rush to that conclusion.

C.   Impact of interpersonal conflict on self and others

1 No evidence of conflict
2 Slight evidence that problems of conflict have hindered the individual in any aspect of personal, social, or occupational life
3 Clear evidence that conflict has hindered personal, social, or occupational adjustment with lowered expectations of future and may also have had a negative impact on others
4 Considerable evidence that the individual and others have suffered failures in personal, social, or occupational aspects of life with a clear negative impact on others
5 Widespread evidence of disruptive life course with inability to achieve good relationships in all areas of personal, social, or occupational life.

- ☐ Score impact of interpersonal conflict

D.   Capacity for mutual understanding

The questioning here can become difficult. In situations where conflict is rife, there is rarely good on one side and bad on the other. The expression 'it takes two to tango' can change to 'it takes two to tangle' very easily. But ownership of negative behaviour is difficult. When I was eight and nine, I liked playing the board game Monopoly. But if you know the game well, you will realise that near the end of the game, it is obvious who is going to win—the player with houses and hotels all over the board—and at this point, if I was losing, I would often have an argument and storm off before finishing the game. I would blame others for the squabble, but everyone knew the real reason. When in an argument one person claims to be completely in the right at all times, you need to ask a few more questions to tease out all the reasons behind the disagreement. You can then score your conclusions:

1 No evidence of any difficulty in accepting and understanding one's own personal functioning
2 Slight evidence of gaps in self-understanding so any difficulties with others are not seen as in any way contributed by the individual
3 Clear evidence that understanding of others is impaired to the extent that the individual is unable to identify the needs and motives of others and so cannot achieve a healthy balance in relationships, but this does not lead to significant malfunction
4 Marked evidence that understanding of others is significantly impaired to the extent that the individual dismisses the needs and motives of others and sees them only in terms of his or her own functioning

5 Very severe mismatch between the individual's own views and those of others so mutual awareness is lacking, and both exploitative and dismissive behaviour aggravate relationships with major ill effects

- ☐ Score capacity for mutual understanding

As an exercise, you can look at the five people we have already described. It would be very difficult to give much in the way of scores to Arthur as he never seems to be in conflict with anyone; Bethany would score in recognising a low level of conflict in her work and appreciate the reasons for it; Callum would also admit to problems in relationships but would quickly turn to alcohol for the reason and not accept his personality as contributing much; Dorothea would give a host of reasons for negative behaviour and probably give equal blame to herself and many others; Eric would have dozens of reasons for being aggressive and paranoid that could be partly attributed to past trauma but in no way could be used to justify his present behaviour.

Nidotherapy

Nidotherapy leaves a negligible memory trace compared with personality disorder but has the advantage of much greater positive connotations. It is a treatment approach that is commonly called transdiagnostic, which means it can be relevant to all mental disorders. But another way of putting this is to say it is non-specific, suggesting it is just an add-on to other interventions that are more focused. Changing your life by leaving the country and taking up a completely new existence can help every form of mental illness if the new environment is more conducive to your needs, but making the change is very difficult to put into operational terms, and it may fail completely if even a relatively minor fault appears in the programme.

In our work in nidotherapy over the years, it has become apparent that attention to the underlying personality structure of the person is a major key to understanding what is likely to help and where failure is more likely. What has also been demonstrated very conclusively is that when a personality disorder gets better, it is often related to environmental change. Time after time, it has been demonstrated that personality development is about 50% determined by your genes and 50% by environment (Jang et al., 1996), but their effects are not independent, and gene-environment interactions can have major effects on behaviour. But the research effort in this area has not been productive in generating new treatments. Research into the treatment of personality disorders has revolved for decades around borderline personality disorder, a condition which we will see many times in this book has been like a moth to the flame for researchers, attracted by the excitement of the heat and light and then getting close enough to be burned with very little to show. It has been known for decades that abuse, especially sexual abuse, in childhood can be a precursor of emotional instability, identity problems, and recurring broken relationships (Herman et al., 1989; Lock et al., 2025), but here, the genetic component has been largely ignored, with most attention being paid to trauma.

What has grown enormously is the science of epigenetics. These are changes in the expression of genes that do not involve any alteration to the genetic code but can be still passed down to another generation. Lifestyle and personality are very important in epigenetics. I am an identical twin, so I and my brother have exactly the same genes. If our environments were the same, as indeed our environments were throughout early life, school, and university, one might expect that our paths would continue to run in parallel. But they have not, and right from the beginning, our teachers and our parents noted we had different personalities. In formal testing at the age of eight, my brother was noted to be very quick on the uptake of new information but did not persist in developing this further, whereas I was slower on uptake but much more methodical and thorough in following things through. These different patterns have consistently been present throughout our lives. Epigenetics was at work at a very young age.

Roy Plomin has commented about this in a similar fashion:

> It was reasonable to assume that the key influences on children's development are those that are shared by children growing up in the same family: their parents' personality and family experiences, the quality of their parents' marital relationship, their parents' educational background and socioeconomic status, the neighbourhood in which they are raised and their parents' attitude to school or to discipline. Yet to the extent that these influences are shared environmentally, they cannot account for individual differences in children's development because the salient environmental influences are non-shared. The message is not that family experiences are unimportant but rather that the relevant experiences are specific to each child in the family, not general to all children in the family.
>
> (Plomin, 2011)

The development of personality is a mix of genetic and epigenetic factors that ensures that no personalities, not even those of identical twins, are the same.

There are two important studies (Caspi et al., 2002; Caspi et al., 2003) that have shown a relationship between genes and environment. The first, taken from a longitudinal study of children from birth to adulthood, showed that those who suffered physical abuse and harsh lives as children were more likely to develop conduct disorder later if they were born with a polymorphism in the monoamine oxidase A (MAOA) gene. The second study suggested that those who had longer versions of the serotonin transporter gene (serotonin being a major brain transmitter) were less likely to develop depression when exposed to stress than those who had the shorter version.

I am not going to go into any depth about the merits of these studies, although they are not immune to criticism, only to point out that personality status was not recorded in either of these studies, and both of these studies focused on negative gene-environment interactions. Virtually no attempt has been made to assess the effect of positive environments. This omission has been noticed by some critics:

> [I]n order to fully understand the role of the environment in the pathophysiology of personality disorders, it will be critical to assess and characterize the effects of the full range of environments (i.e., from highly enriched or positive to highly deprived or negative).
>
> (Bulbena-Cabre et al., 2018)

Why nidotherapy is of special value in connection with personality

Personality is the driver behind our lives. Although many believe that chance is much more important and that many of the decisions we make and their outcomes are randomly determined, what brings all of these to fruition is our personalities. And how we respond to pressures in life is not just determined by a rogue gene or two; it is determined by a combination of intellectual and personal factors that together are influenced by many genes and many environments. So throughout our lives, we, our personalities, and the many genes underlying them are sparring with the environment in finding the most fruitful matches. When these do not turn out well, we become distressed and mentally unwell. A much more robust set of findings than the Caspi studies is clear evidence that if you have a personality disorder, you are much less likely to respond to treatment for a common condition such as depression or anxiety than if your personality is stable (Newton-Howes et al., 2006; Newton-Howes et al., 2014; Skodol et al., 2014; Goddard et al., 2015).

What does this tell us about the influence of personality on health? It is not an odd gene or two that keeps you unwell when others have different genes so they get better. Your personality structure is what lies behind the persistence of common mental health problems, and this persistence is shown with all treatments. It is also quite possible that your personality, rumbling away in the background, is the reason some people are more vulnerable to both onset and relapse of mental disorder and might be the main precipitant of most clinical problems (Tyrer, 2015).

Nidotherapy takes this subject into the positive arena. If the mix of your personality and environment is making you unwell, the right way to tackle it is to change the environment from a negative to a positive one. Because we cannot create positive environments with a wave of a wand, we have to nurture and develop them. Sometimes we know what we need to do to make the environment a positive one, but often we don't, at least at first, and this is where nidotherapy comes in handy.

But changing environments is what healthy people do all the time when they feel dissatisfied with their present situations. We change our jobs when we realise they are unfulfilling, we change partners when the real person appears after the gloss, we change our accommodation when we need more space, and we change our leisure pursuits from energetic team games to golf when our bones begin to creak. So all this can be called nidotherapy, as we are changing our environments to have a greater degree of satisfaction.

When we first introduced nidotherapy to an unsuspecting psychiatric public, there was a large sigh of condescension—it's what we do all the time in our work; what's new? But most practitioners rarely practise nidotherapy as a craft, a careful examination of a difficult environmental problem that cannot be solved alone but which needs help in achieving the right change. So when somebody who is mentally unwell because they have nowhere to live, cannot separate from a controlling spouse or start a new career from scratch, or is looking after a dementing relative, what does the average practitioner do? Nothing, apart from soft words of sympathy or occasionally a referral to another agency.

Nobody is expecting every mental health professional to be a Mother Theresa, tending to everybody in a neighbourhood without question, but when it is apparent that the environmental problems needing to be solved are closely related to aspects of the personality then, I argue, it is an appropriate professional task to address these needs in some way. This is where adaptation comes in. We need to match the personality both to the need and to the environment concerned. This can sometimes be straightforward— a homeless person needs accommodation, not a shoulder to cry on—but often, it is much more complicated. It is only by applying the principles of adaptation that the right environment, often a highly specialised environment with many components, is going to be the answer. And when it is chosen correctly, mental health improves.

Our research team has been involved in a follow-up of people with the common mental disorders of anxiety and depression who presented at outpatient clinics in Nottingham in the early 1980s. They received a great deal of conventional treatment over this 30-year period, but after this time, only a few had recovered; most had continued to have symptoms and were no better than when they started. But there were exceptions. In analysing the environmental changes that had taken place over follow-up, we were quite surprised. It was only those patients who had experienced marked positive environmental changes who had really got better (Tyrer et al., 2024).

We have no idea how many of these changes were a consequence of nidotherapy, but we suspect there would have been many more recoveries had we been practising this approach over the period of follow-up (most of which was completely independent of the follow-up team). We also found that those with personality disorder at baseline assessment had significantly fewer positive changes that those without personality problems (Tyrer et al., 2024). The rest of this book attempts to show how this finding can be reversed, not only by professionals in mental health but also with added input from lay people who understand the principles of nidotherapy and can use them in practice.

References

Ahmed Z & Tyrer P (2024). The benefits and hazards of psychodrama in the management of mental illness: qualitative study linked to nidotherapy. *BJPsych Bulletin*, 1–5. https://doi.org/10.1192/bjb.2024.57.

Akerman G, Needs A, & Bainbridge C (eds). (2018). *Transforming Environments and Rehabilitation: A Guide for Practitioners in Forensic Settings and Criminal Justice.* Abingdon: Routledge.

Bach B, Brown TA, Mulder RT, Newton-Howes G, Simonsen E, & Sellbom M (2021). Development and initial evaluation of the ICD-11 personality disorder severity scale: PDS-ICD–11. *Personality and Mental Health*, 15, 223–236.

Bateman AW (2011). Throwing the baby out with the bathwater? [Commentary]. *Personality and Mental Health*, 5, 274–280.

Boyle H & Johnstone L (2020). *A Straight Talking Introduction to the Power Threat Meaning Framework: An Alternative to Psychiatric Diagnosis.* PCCS Books.

Bulbena-Cabre A, Bassir Nia A, & Perez-Rodriguez MM (2018). Current knowledge on gene-environment Interactions in personality disorders: an update. *Current Psychiatry Reports*, 20, 74.

Caspi A, McClay J, Moffitt TE, Mill J, Martin J, Craig IW, et al. (2002). Role of genotype in the cycle of violence in maltreated children. *Science*, 297, 851–854.

Caspi A, Sugden K, Moffitt TE, Taylor A, Craig IW, Harrington H, et al. (2003). Influence of life stress on depression: moderation by a polymorphism in the 5-HTT gene. *Science*, 301, 386–389.

Davidson K (2011). Changing the classification of personality disorders—an ICD-11 proposal that goes too far? [Editorial]. *Personality and Mental Health*, 5, 243–245.

Fry S (2018). Foreword. In: P Tyrer (ed.), *Taming the Beast Within: Shredding the Stereotypes of Personality Disorder.* Sheldon Press.

Goddard E, Wingrove J, & Moran P (2015). The impact of comorbid personality difficulties on response to IAPT treatment for depression and anxiety. *Behaviour Research and Therapy*, 73, 1–7.

Herman JL, Perry JC, & van der Kolk BA (1989). Childhood trauma in borderline personality disorder. *American Journal of Psychiatry*, 146, 490–495.

Jang KL, Livesley WJ, Vernon PA, & Jackson DN (1996). Heritability of personality disorder traits: a twin study. *Acta Psychiatrica Scandinavica*, 94, 438–444.

Kim Y-R, Tyrer P, & Hwang S-T (2021). Personality Assessment Questionnaire for ICD-11 personality trait domains: development and testing. *Personality and Mental Health*, 15, 58–71.

Kotov R, Krueger RF, Watson D, Achenbach TM, Althoff RR, Bagby RM, et al. (2017). The Hierarchical Taxonomy of Psychopathology (HiTOP): a dimensional alternative to traditional nosologies. *Journal of Abnormal Psychology*, 126, 454–477.

Lock J, Yang M, & Tyrer P (2025). Establishing the relationship between history of childhood trauma and personality disorder using the ICD-11 classification system. *Personality and Mental Health*, 19, e1648.

Loranger AW, Sartorius N, Andreoli A, Berger P, Buchheim P, Channabasavanna SM, et al. (1994). The International Personality Disorder Examination. The World Health Organization/Alcohol, Drug Abuse, and Mental Health Administration international pilot study of personality disorders. *Archives of General Psychiatry*, 51, 215–224.

Moran P, Leese M, Lee T, Walters P, Thornicroft G, & Mann A (2003). Standardised Assessment of Personality—Abbreviated Scale (SAPAS): preliminary validation of a brief screen for personality disorder. *British Journal of Psychiatry*, 183, 228–232.

Newton-Howes G, Tyrer P, & Johnson T (2006). Personality disorder and the outcome of depression: a meta-analysis of published studies. *British Journal of Psychiatry*, 188, 13–20.

Newton-Howes G, Tyrer P, Johnson T, Mulder R, Kool S, Dekker J, et al. (2014). Influence of personality on the outcome of treatment in depression: systematic review and meta-analysis. *Journal of Personality Disorders*, 28, 577–593.

Olajide K, Munjiza J, Moran P, O'Connell L, Newton-Howes G, Bassett P, Gbolagade A, et al. (2018). Development and psychometric properties of the Standardized Assessment of Severity of Personality Disorder (SASPD). *Journal of Personality Disorders*, 32, 44–56.

Oltmanns JR & Widiger TA (2018). A self-report measure for the ICD-11 dimensional trait model proposal: The personality inventory for ICD-11. *Psychological Assessment*, 30, 154–169.

Owen D (2008). Hubris syndrome. *Clinical Medicine*, 8, 428–432.

Owen D (2012). *The Hubris Syndrome: Bush, Blair and the Intoxication of Power*. Methuen.

Plomin R (2011). Commentary: why are children in the same family so different? non-shared environment three decades later. *International Journal of Epidemiology*, 40, 582–592.

Ranger M, Tyrer P, Miloseska K, Fourie H, Khaleel I, North B, et al. (2009). Cost-effectiveness of nidotherapy for comorbid personality disorder and severe mental illness: randomized controlled trial. *Epidemiologia e Psichiatria Sociale*, 18, 128–136.

Skodol AE, Geier T, Grant BF, & Hasin DS (2014). Personality disorders and the persistence of anxiety disorders in a nationally representative sample. *Depression and Anxiety*, 31, 721–728.

Spears B, Tyrer H, & Tyrer P (2017). Nidotherapy in the successful management of comorbid depressive and personality disorder. *Personality and Mental Health*, 11, 344–350.

Spencer S-J, Rutter D, & Tyrer P (2010). Integration of nidotherapy into the management of mental illness and antisocial personality: a qualitative study. *International Journal of Social Psychiatry*, 56, 50–59.

Svrakic DM, Lecic-Tosevski D, & Divac-Jovanovic M (2009). DSM axis II: personality disorders or adaptation disorders? *Current Opinion in Psychiatry*, 22, 111–117.

Tyrer P (2009). *Nidotherapy: Harmonising the Environment with the Patient*. London: RCPsych Press.

Tyrer P (2015). Personality dysfunction is the cause of recurrent non-cognitive mental disorder: a testable hypothesis. *Personality and Mental Health*, 9, 1–7.

Tyrer P (2018). *Taming the Beast Within: Shredding the Stereotypes of Personality Disorder*. London: Sheldon Press.

Tyrer P & Bajaj P (2005). Nidotherapy: making the environment do the therapeutic work. *Advances in Psychiatric Treatment*, 11, 232–238.

Tyrer P, Crawford M, Mulder RT, Blashfield R, Farnam A, Fossati A, et al. (2011). The rationale for the reclassification of personality disorder in the 11th revision of the International Classification of Diseases (ICD-11). *Personality and Mental Health*, 5, 246–259.

Tyrer P, Duggan C, Yang M, & Tyrer H (2024). The effect of environmental change, planned and unplanned life events on the long-term outcome of common mental disorders. *Social Psychiatry and Psychiatric Epidemiology*, 59, 1587–1598.

Tyrer P & Mulder R (2022). *Personality Disorder: From Evidence to Understanding*. Cambridge University Press.

Tyrer P, Sensky T, & Mitchard S (2003). The principles of nidotherapy in the treatment of persistent mental and personality disorders. *Psychotherapy and Psychosomatics*, 72, 350–356.

Tyrer P, Tarabi SA, Bassett P, Liedtka N, Hall R, Nagar J, et al. (2017). Nidotherapy compared with enhanced care programme approach training for adults with aggressive challenging behaviour and intellectual disability (NIDABID): cluster-randomised controlled trial. *Journal of Intellectual Disability Research*, 61, 521–531.

Tyrer P & Tyrer H (2018). *Nidotherapy: Harmonising the Environment with the Patient* (2nd edition). Cambridge: Cambridge University Press.

World Health Organisation (2024). *Clinical Descriptions and Diagnostic Requirements for ICD-11 Mental, Behavioural and Neurodevelopmental Disorders*. WHO: Geneva.

Chapter 2

Why ICD-11 helps facilitate treatment of personality disorder

A good postal system has a highly efficient way of getting letters and other documents to the right addresses. It used to be done by hand but is now automatic. A good diagnostic system should be equally efficient. Many such systems in general medicine follow the post office model. If you fall over and fracture your femur, you will go into the hip replacement box for your care. It would be a major error if you were sent to a knee replacement service instead.

We do not yet have efficient postbox equivalents in psychiatry, and as a consequence, all diagnoses have to be provisional. To use the postal equivalent, we are in a land where we know most people live, but there are no such thing as addresses, and so we only have a vague idea where to deliver our letters. We therefore rely on our intrepid postman to make the right decisions.

The diagnosis of personality disorder is in equivalent terrain. But this is not the only problem. Because some people feel the subject is so grossly stigmatised, they argue that the diagnosis should be removed altogether and replaced by another set of words (see the last chapter of this book). One option that has attracted a lot of attention recently is that of complex emotional needs (Ledden et al., 2022), said to be a preferred working term for people who have a 'personality disorder' diagnosis or comparable needs. This is not an answer to the problem; the right answer is to address the stigma and not to introduce a mushy word sandwich that only confuses by making the condition almost universal—don't we all have complex emotional needs? (Porter et al., 2025).

ICD-11 removes stigma from personality disorder

Stigma in mental health is present when a subject generates a negative attitude or idea that implies social disapproval. The social disapproval attached to personality disorder need not be repeated again here, but I argue in this chapter and in the last chapter of this book that social disapproval of a

DOI: 10.4324/9781003560630-2

mental disorder is not removed by shouting 'stigma' at every street corner, but will be reduced and may even disappear once you have a successful straightforward form of management. It also disappears once a condition is recognised as being possessed by everyone. One of the most respected psychiatrists of the 20th century was Aubrey Lewis, who was mainly responsible for making the subject a proper academic discipline. He wrote a paper on depression in 1936, 'Melancholia: A Clinical Survey of Depressive States. Note the title: 'Melancholia'. It was a very long article, over 100 pages (no editor would allow that today), and described in detail the symptoms of 61 patients with depression. But it changed attitudes. Before this time, melancholia and mania were two severe conditions of insanity, regarded as beyond the pale of help or recovery. By teasing out all the different symptoms of depression, Lewis brought the subject into the light of common parlance. Many people had depression; it was not insanity, it fluctuated and was seldom permanent, and the stigma of melancholia gradually ebbed away. The same should apply to personality disorder; we all have a bit of it, and it affects all our relationships. We should be proud of our personality diversity and not allow self-stigma, the belief that there is something unworthy and shameful in us if we acknowledge the presence of a personality problem.

The more murky a diagnosis, the more it is subject to stigma, as ignorance leads to fear and suspicion that the diagnosis is only given in order to reject. Compared with other diagnoses in psychiatry, personality disorder is in the fourth division of acceptability. Some years ago, that excellent pioneer of psychiatric classification Robert (Bob) Kendell bluntly castigated the state of knowledge of personality disorder:

> There is also a glaring need for a better classification of personality disorders and for more long-term follow-up studies of representative samples, derived from community rather than clinical populations, to answer basic questions about the extent, nature and time course of the handicaps associated with different types of personality disorder.
>
> (Kendell, 2002, p. 113)

We still have some way to go, but I argue that the ICD-11 classification of personality disorder will help answer most of these questions. It will need considerable time, partly because good studies in this area need long-term follow-up.

The International Classification of Diseases was launched in Paris in 1900 and has been revised every few years since. The tenth revision (ICD-10) was introduced in 1990 and came into effect in 1993. At that time, personality disorder was a peripheral subject in psychiatry, and many clinicians did not consider it a mental disorder at all. Yet it was included in the classification of mental and behavioural disorders with the summary description that had been part of the definition for most previous ICD versions: 'deeply ingrained and enduring behaviour patterns, manifesting as inflexible responses to a broad range of personal and social situations' (World Health Organisation, 1992). Note the 'deeply ingrained' and 'inflexible responses', words designed to stress that these were disorders that were not going to get better. But these words were all repeated from previous versions. At that time, nobody had carried out research into the long-term persistence of personality disorder; when that was done, it was shown to be a very unstable condition (Paris, 2003; Yang et al., 2022), so 'ingrained' is no longer used as an adjective in ICD-11; 'inflexible' is confined mainly to descriptions of autism (World Health Organisation, 2024); and, when attached to personality disorder, it now receives an option in brackets (see p. 14, Chapter 1).

ICD-10 then went on to list 'specific personality disorders'. These immediately attracted so much attention that everyone forgot about the general description and went directly for the specifics of paranoid, schizoid, dissocial, emotionally unstable, histrionic, anankastic, anxious, and dependent personality disorders. Clinicians also had the option of diagnosing eccentric, haltlose (combination of antisocial and histrionic), immature, narcissistic, passive aggressive, and psychoneurotic personality disorders. Each of these disorders had a precise description. The emotionally unstable group was separated into two: the impulsive type was characterised by reckless unexpected behaviour, liability to outbursts of anger, difficulty in maintaining any course of action, and unstable mood, and the borderline type was characterised by disturbances in self-image, the tendency to become involved in intensely unstable relationships, excessive efforts to avoid abandonment, recurrent threats or acts of self harm, and chronic feelings of emptiness.

These terms will be mentioned elsewhere in this book, but it is important that in ICD-11, these categories no longer exist as diagnoses. The only one that has persisted is borderline, but that only owes its existence to a campaign by those who have invested a great deal of time and energy into investigating this condition. In order to maintain continuity, there is now a 'pattern specifier' in the diagnostic system for borderline, but it is not a diagnosis and not part of the central classification.

What is clear is that personality problems do not disappear overnight and tend to persist longer than other conditions, but there are exceptions, many linked to environmental change, that you will encounter later in this book.

Why were the categories abolished in ICD-11?

There were two good reasons why categories of personality disorder were abolished in ICD-11. The first was a simple one of utility. No diagnosis, no matter how accurate and precise, is of value if it is never used. All the categories listed earlier were ignored apart from two, the borderline sub-division of emotionally unstable personality disorder and dissocial, also called antisocial or psychopathic personality disorder. The rest just disappeared into oblivion, especially the impulsive form of emotionally unstable personality disorder, which, to my knowledge, has never been described in a research paper. The second reason is a scientific one. When researchers made a special effort to diagnose personality disorder in different population groups, they found that there was a very marked overlap between the different categories. Often these were so difficult to disentangle that the clinician could make a diagnosis of mixed personality disorder or, in the American equivalent, DSM, allow a combined personality disorder-not otherwise specified (PD-NOS).

So what became clear was that the representation of personality abnormality in clinical practice was completely unlike the classification system that existed to code it (Tyrer & Johnson, 1996). The system was broken, and the main reason was that nobody had challenged the original classification of personality disorder devised by Kurt Schneider, a German psychiatrist of considerable distinction, who had described the categories of personality disorder in 1923 in exactly the same form that they subsequently were listed in ICD-10 (Schneider, 1923). The other culprit was the American system, DSM-III, which revolutionised psychiatric classification in 1980 but still followed the same system as Schneider in describing a similar set of categories. One that caused a great deal of interest was passive aggressive personality disorder, but this category seemed to arise from the frustration of psychoanalysts whose patients were very slow in paying for their treatment.

The fundamental problem was that the categories of personality disorder were cartoon figures, not real people. They were fun, but not real. So we have the narcissistic Jessica Rabbit ('I'm not bad; I'm just drawn that way'); Bugs Bunny, the borderline ('I'll be scared later. Right now I'm too mad'); Charlie Brown, the neurotic avoidant ('Worrying won't stop the bad things from happening; it just stops you enjoying the good'); Mr Burns, the antisocial controlling boss ('You've made a powerful enemy today, my friend'); and Eeyore, the depressive, isolated donkey ('We can't all, and some of us don't'). They are lovable, but real people, as Jessica Rabbit would emphasise, are not drawn that way. They are fun to write about—that's where Donald Trump gets a lot of his oxygen—but they are the stuff of fantasy.

Across the Atlantic, some years before the introduction of ICD-10, the American psychiatric equivalent of ICD, the Diagnostic and Statistical

Manual of Mental Disorders (DSM-III-R) (1987) realised that this pot-pourri of different diagnoses was not likely to be particularly helpful and so introduced the concept of three clusters of personality disturbance. The three clusters, introduced without any evidence of their accuracy or value, were the odd, eccentric cluster (Cluster A); the dramatic, erratic cluster (Cluster B); and the anxious, fearful cluster (Cluster C). Cluster A included the paranoid, schizoid, and schizotypal personalities; Cluster B included the antisocial borderline histrionic and narcissistic personalities; and Cluster C had the avoidant, dependent, and compulsive personalities. Although to some, this just looked like moving the deck chairs around on a sinking ship, it did at least shorten the list of abnormal personalities.

The one advantage of having an international classification system, no matter how defective, is that the frequency of disorders can be evaluated in epidemiological studies across the world. The results of two recent reviews, preceding the new ICD-11 classification, are shown in Table 2.1.

The variation in these figures illustrates that the assessment of personality disorder is far from precise, but the data are still very useful. The first thing to notice is the big difference between the prevalence of personality disorders in high-income countries and those in low-income countries (Winsper et al., 2020). This is unlikely to be an error of measurement and suggests that one of the disadvantages of Western civilisation has been the promotion of personality disturbance. Why should this be? As countries become more Westernised, there is a greater trend to individualism and independence. This leads to a change in relationships.

Achieving the cultural goal of independence requires construing one-self as an individual whose behavior is organized and made meaning-ful primarily by reference to one's own internal repertoire of thoughts,

Table 2.1 Prevalence of personality disorder across the world, separated by high and low income countries (Volkert et al., 2018; Winsper et al., 2020)

Data source	All personality disorders	Cluster A prevalence (%)	Cluster B prevalence (%)	Cluster C prevalence (%)
Volkert et al., 2018 (world)	12.2	7.2	5.5	6.7
Winsper et al., 2020 (world)	7.8	3.8	2.8	5.0
Winsper (high-income countries)	9.6	4.2	3.7	6.6
Winsper (low-income countries)	4.3	3.4	1.5	3.3

feelings, and action, rather than by reference to the thoughts, feelings, and actions of others.

(Markus & Kitayama, 1991, p. 226)

This is in contrast to the collectivist or interdependent self, in which

[T]he relationship between the self and others features the person not as separate from the social context but as more connected and less differentiated from others. People are motivated to find a way to fit in with relevant others, to fulfil and create obligation, and in general to become part of various interpersonal relationships. Unlike the independent self, the significant features of the self according to this construal are to be found in the interdependent and thus, in the more public components of the self.

(Markus & Kitayama, 1991, p. 227)

It is reasonable to conclude that those with personality problems are more likely to succeed and be accepted in a collectivist societal framework. Those with antisocial behaviour who are socially excluded may still have difficulties, but most of those who deviate from the norm are more likely to be embraced and brought back into the fold. There is also greater tolerance of diversity. One of the most radical ways by which people can adapt to personality difficulties is to move from an individualist society to a collectivist one. Robert Louis Stevenson did this when he left Scotland and other Western countries and settled in Samoa, where his wilder moments were tempered by a close relationship with the islanders there, a place where he is still revered. 'We are all travellers in the wilderness of this world, and the best we can find in our travels is an honest friend'.

The second striking piece of information in Table 2.1 is the high prevalence of Cluster A and C disorders compared with Cluster B. This is not what you would expect from looking at the literature on personality disorder, where almost everything seems to refer to borderline. The pooled prevalence figures for borderline personality disorder were 1.8% (Winsper) and 1.9% (Volkert), so accounting for under a quarter of the total. The great majority of people with personality disorders do not seek treatment because they do not want their personalities altered (Type R or treatment-resisting personalities) (Tyrer et al., 2003), or, if they do, nothing is available to help them. The major failure of clinical practice in the management of personality disorders has been the almost-total neglect of personality problems outside the borderline group in ordinary clinical practice and the antisocial group in forensic settings. Later chapters in this book try to redress the balance.

Why ICD-11 has improved understanding

The ICD-11 classification bothered many clinicians when it was first introduced. It was regarded as too radical, premature, insufficiently based on research data, and an example of 'medical expansionism'. This was understandable; big changes to a standard, familiar process scare many and irritate others, but over the course of the last 15 years, it has achieved wide acceptance and approval (Bach & First, 2018; Aluja et al., 2022; Bach & Mulder, 2022; Hualparuca-Olivera et al., 2024; Bangash, 2022, 2024). This approval covers several areas—its links to the big five factors of normal personality (Mccrae & Costa, 1984), its ease of use (Bach & First, 2018), its value in child and adolescent psychiatry (Wilkinson, 2022; Pan & Wang, 2024), and its acceptance across the range of psychodynamic and clinical practice (Blüml & Doering, 2021).

The most important consequence of this is that the classification is likely to be used in common clinical practice, in contrast to ICD-10, which was virtually ignored except for the diagnosis of borderline (emotionally unstable) and antisocial (dissocial) personality disorders. It is also likely that the different levels of personality disturbance can be identified relatively easily. What happened in the use of ICD-10 was that only when personality disorder became prominent (i.e., at least moderately severe) was it considered in diagnostic terms; the greater range, including personality difficulty, will help both clinical practice and research. In particular, personality difficulty, being a completely new classification item in personality disturbance, can be studied more closely to see whether its high frequency in prevalence studies is associated with greater social dysfunction and psychiatric disturbance. Some of the initial data suggest that this may be the case (Karukivi et al., 2017; Tyrer et al., 2022).

Another advantage of the ICD-11 classification is that it does not restrict the onset of diagnosis to early adult life. If personality disturbance is shown for two years or more (see Chapter 1, p. 8), it can be diagnosed as personality disorder. This allows the diagnosis to be made in adolescence (Chanen et al., 2008; Pan & Wang, 2024) and also in old age for the first time (Penders et al., 2020; Bangash, 2022).

There has been a great deal of controversy over the diagnosis of personality disorder in young people. In the past it was very rarely diagnosed as neither of the two classifications, ICD and DSM, allowed the diagnosis in the young (Laurenssen et al., 2013). But then a series of studies and reviews prompted a rethink (Chanen et al., 2008, 2020; Pan & Wang, 2024). Despite this, there is considerable reluctance to use the diagnosis in adolescence, and the need to involve the patient more in reaching the diagnosis has been strongly emphasised (Papadopoullos et al., 2022). Many feel that once the diagnosis of personality disorder has been made in adolescence, it will be affixed for life unfairly. It is absolutely true that personality disorder diagnosed in adolescence is much more likely to disappear in adulthood than if it is diagnosed later (Cohen et al., 2005) although, in the short term, it may be associated with greater pathology (Ayodeji et al., 2015). The likely transience of personality disorder should always be stressed if it is diagnosed in the young.

The other great advantage of ICD-11 is that it allows treatment to be graded in intensity for each level of personality disturbance. At present, using the ICD and DSM diagnostic systems, there is a simple cut-off between no personality disturbance and personality disorder with no indication of severity. A small proportion of these people can be treated with highly intensive treatments, but we do not know at what level of severity they would be most helpful. This is a very unhelpful set of circumstances and explains much of the frustration that patients have about receiving treatment.

Once ICD-11 has been properly implemented, we will be able to study whether much shorter forms of psychological treatment may be at least equally effective for the less severe personality disorders (e.g., structured psychological support, currently being assessed in a large trial of over 300 subjects (Crawford et al., 2020). The same may apply to other treatments such as drug prescription and the many briefer forms of psychological treatment, including social prescribing, that might well be effective in mild personality disorder and associated Galenic syndromes.

Yet another advantage of the ICD-11 system is that it allows all types of personality disturbance to be considered in the diagnosis. This is because it is possible to qualify the severity of personality disturbance with any number of the five domain traits that are discussed in the next chapter. When personality disturbance gets more severe, more of these domain traits are involved, and so adaptive strategies for dealing with combined conditions can readily be tested. This is not possible with the ICD-10 structure.

Because there are several hundred ways of classifying personality disorder using the combination of severity and domain trait structure, it is likely that only a few combinations will dominate clinical practice, and these are the ones that will require close scrutiny.

Much more needs to be told about the importance of personality difficulty in both short- and long-term outcome of personality disturbance. This is likely to be of particular value in child and adolescent psychiatry. At present, there is considerable alarm, if that is not too strong a word, about the great increase in diagnosis of autism spectrum and attention deficit hyperactivity disorder (ADHD). These findings are unlikely to represent a genuine increase in the number of these disorders, and much of it has been generated by social media and loose diagnostic practice, possibly accentuated by the recent COVID-19 pandemic. It is likely that a significant proportion of the adolescents diagnosed with these disorders have temporary personality disturbance associated with difficulties in schooling and parental supervision. If this is indeed the case, then it would be much better for these children to be helped by environmental changes such as nidotherapy instead of being subjected to more intensive treatments and the problems associated with their long-term sequelae.

I have argued for many years that good psychiatric practice involves making both a mental state assessment and a personality one. Although many pay lip service to this policy, it is seldom applied in practice. What is much more common is for patients that have no personality assessment at first that is worthy of the name, and then, at a later date, when they have failed to respond to the treatment given, a further assessment is made and the diagnosis of personality disorder added retrospectively. This is not only bad practice but also unfairly stigmatises personality disorder. The assumption that having a personality disorder or any form of personality disturbance leads to a worse outcome for mental disorders may sometimes be true but certainly not always. In a very large randomised controlled trial of cognitive behaviour therapy in medical patients with health anxiety, we found that those with personality disorder, particularly when anxious and dependent features were prominent, had a better outcome than those without personality problems, and these differences persisted up to eight years after initial treatment (with no booster sessions after the first few months) (Sanatinia et al., 2016; Tyrer et al., 2021).

The place of nidotherapy will also become clearer once the ICD-11 system is fully operational. If practitioners can become experienced in diagnosing both mental state and personality problems, then the place of environmental change in management becomes much clearer. Instead of personality disorder being diagnosed in retrospect, often quite wrongly, any personality difficulties at any level of severity can be identified earlier on in treatment and adaptive interventions made.

Case example

A young man was seen following a serious suicidal episode when driving his car that was prevented at the last moment. He had become gradually more depressed over the previous three years because he was uncertain about his occupational future and had a girl-friend with whom relations were stormy. Assessment of his personality showed that he had a history of making impulsive decisions when under stress, and most of these had turned out very badly. He responded very well to standard antidepressant drug therapy, and in the management of his impulsive nature, it was felt valuable to promote his interest in acting. He took part in several plays, one of which was supported by an external grant, and he played the part of a detective in a murder plot. As his confidence increased, he was able to stop his antidepressants and continue his acting successfully so his self-esteem improved. This led him, almost inexorably, toward the practice of law as a profession. He is now well established in a legal role and is looking forward to real-life courtroom drama in the future.

This example illustrates the increased breadth of treating a mental illness (depression) with awareness of personality (impulsiveness and need for drama) in a combined way. In nidotherapy we often use drama as a way of promoting personality strengths and self-esteem, and it has largely been successful (Mansell et al., 2024), provided all are aware of the potential negative aspects of public performance (Ahmed & Tyrer, 2024). Clearly there could have been many other ways of helping this young man move toward a positive future, but the ability to both harness his personality characteristics and provide standard treatment for depression has led to a much better outcome that might otherwise have been expected.

It is also mutually reinforcing. Knowing that a course of treatment for depression is likely to be self-limited because the other positive life events are in place is a much more satisfactory outcome than merely treating the depression and discharging the patient with no clear idea of what led the patient to seek treatment.

This example indicates the subtle aspects of personality that can facilitate treatment strategies in psychiatry. The constant awareness of the personality problem, even though present at the low level of personality difficulty, helped all aspects of the management of this young man and may have been the main element behind a successful new career, an example of occupational nidotherapy. But the case also illustrates that the simple level of personality disturbance is not enough for understanding; it also requires assessment of the domain traits that lie behind each level.

References

Ahmed Z & Tyrer P (2024). The benefits and hazards of psychodrama in the management of mental illness: qualitative study linked to nidotherapy. *BJPsych Bulletin*. https://doi.org/10.11.1192/bjb/2024.57.

Aluja A, Sorrel MA, García LF, Garcí O, & Gutierrez F (2022). Factor convergence and predictive analysis of the five factor and alternative five factor personality models with the five-factor personality inventory for ICD-11 (FFiCD). *Journal of Personality Disorders*, 36, 296–319.

Ayodeji E, Green J, Roberts C, Trainor G, Rothwell J, Woodham A, et al. (2015). The influence of personality disorder on outcome in adolescent self-harm. *British Journal of Psychiatry*, 207, 313–319.

Bach B & First MB (2018). Application of the ICD-11 classification of personality disorders. *BMC Psychiatry*, 18, 351.

Bach B & Mulder RT (2022). Clinical implications of ICD-11 for diagnosing and treating personality disorders. *Current Psychiatry Reports*, 24, 553–563.

Bangash A (2022). Late life personality disorders: problems in assessment and management. *Personality and Mental Health*, 16, 155–159.

Bangash A (2024). Personality difficulty: a useful addition to the literature on personality disturbance. *Personality and Mental Health*, 18, 435–437.

Blüml V & Doering S (2021). ICD-11 personality disorders: a psychodynamic perspective on personality functioning. *Frontiers in Psychiatry*, 12, 654026.

Chanen AM, Jackson HJ, Mccutcheon LK, Jovev M, Dudgeon P, Yuen HP, et al. (2008). Early intervention for adolescents with borderline personality disorder using cognitive analytic therapy: randomised controlled trial. *British Journal of Psychiatry*, 193, 477–484.

Chanen AM, Nicol K, Betts JK, & Thompson KN (2020). Diagnosis and treatment of borderline personality disorder in young people. *Current Psychiatry Reports*, 22, 25.

Cohen P, Crawford TN, Johnson JG, & Kasen S (2005). The children in the community study of developmental course of personality disorder. *Journal of Personality Disorders*, 19, 466–486.

Crawford MJ, Thana L, Parker J, Turner O, Carney A, McMurran M, et al. (2020). Structured psychological support for people with personality disorder: feasibility randomised controlled trial of a low-intensity intervention. *BJPsych Open*, 6, e25.

Hualparuca-Olivera L, Caycho-Rodríguez T, Torales J, Ramos-Vera C, Ramos-Campos D, Córdova-Gónzalez L, et al. (2024). Internal consistency of measures for ICD-11 personality disorder severity and traits: a systematic review and meta-analysis. *Personality and Mental Health*, 18, 357–368.

Karukivi M, Vahlberg T, Horjamo K, Nevalainen M, & Korkeila J (2017). Clinical importance of personality difficulties: diagnostically sub-threshold personality disorders. *BMC Psychiatry*, 17, 16.

Kendell RE (2002). The distinction between personality disorder and mental illness. *British Journal of Psychiatry*, 180, 110–115.

Laurenssen EM, Hutsebaut J, Feenstra DJ, Van Busschbach JJ, & Luyten P (2013). Diagnosis of personality disorders in adolescents: a study among psychologists. *Child and Adolescent Psychiatry and Mental Health*, 7, 3.

Ledden S, Rains LS, Schlief M, Barnett P, Ching BCF, Hallam B, et al., C. E. N. Mental Health Policy Research Unit Group (2022). Current state of the evidence on community treatments for people with complex emotional needs: a scoping review. *BMC Psychiatry*, 22, 589.

Lewis A (1936). Melancholia: a clinical survey of depressive states. *Journal of Mental Science*, 80, 277–378.

Mansell C, Yang M, & Tyrer P (2024). Effect of drama training on self-esteem and personality strengths: a feasibility case control study of nidotherapy. *International Journal of Social Psychiatry*, 70, 899–903.

Markus HR & Kitayama S (1991). Culture and the self: implications for cognition, emotion and motivation *Psychological Review*, 98, 224–253.

McCrae RR & Costa PT, Jr (1984). *Emerging Lives, Enduring Dispositions: Personality in Adulthood*. Boston, MA: Little, Brown and Co.

Pan B & Wang W (2024). Practical implications of ICD-11 personality disorder classifications. *BMC Psychiatry*, 24, 191.

Papadopoullos R, Fisher P, Leddy A, Maxwell S, & Hodgekins J (2022). Diagnosis and dilemma: clinician experiences of the use of 'borderline personality disorder' diagnosis in children and adolescents. *Personality and Mental Health*, 16, 300–308.

Paris J (2003). Personality disorders over time: precursors, course and outcome. *Journal of Personality Disorders*, 17, 479–488.

Penders KAP, Peeters IGP, Metsemakers JFM, & van Alphen SPJ (2020). Personality disorders in older adults: a review of epidemiology, assessment, and treatment. *Current Psychiatry Reports*, 22, 14.

Porter H, Edwards B, Head N, & Smith J (2025). A brief critique of the pseudo-diagnosis 'complex emotional needs'. *The British Journal of Psychiatry*, 1–3. https://doi.org/10.1192/bjp.2024.291.

Sanatinia R, Wang D, Tyrer P, Tyrer H, Cooper S, Crawford M, et al. (2016). The impact of personality status on the cost and outcomes of cognitive behaviour therapy for health anxiety. *British Journal of Psychiatry*, 209, 244–250.

Schneider K (1923). *Die Psychopathischen Persönlichkeiten*. Leipzig & Wien: Franz Deuticke.

Tyrer P & Johnson T (1996). Establishing the severity of personality disorder. *American Journal of Psychiatry*, 153, 1593–1597.

Tyrer P, Mitchard S, Methuen C, & Ranger M (2003). Treatment-rejecting and treatment-seeking personality disorders: Type R and Type S. *Journal of Personality Disorders*, 17, 265–270.

Tyrer P, Tyrer H, Johnson T, & Yang M. (2022). Thirty-year outcome of anxiety and depressive disorders and personality status: comprehensive evaluation of mixed symptoms and the general neurotic syndrome in the follow-up of a randomised controlled trial. *Psychological Medicine*, 52, 3999–4008.

Tyrer P, Wang D, Tyrer H, Crawford M, Loebenberg G, Cooper S, Barrett B, & Sanatinia R (2021). Influence of apparently negative personality characteristics on the long-term outcome of health anxiety: secondary analysis of a randomised controlled trial. *Personality and Mental Health*, 15, 72–78.

Volkert J, Gablonski TC, & Rabung S (2018). Prevalence of personality disorders in the general adult population in Western countries: systematic review and meta-analysis. *British Journal of Psychiatry*, 213, 709–715.

Wilkinson SR (2022). Diagnosis on the way out—personality on the way in? priorities in treatment in child and adolescent psychiatry. *Clinics in Child Psychology and Psychiatry*, 27, 504–514.

Winsper C, Bilgin A, Thompson A, Marwaha S, Chanen AM, Singh SP, et al. (2020). The prevalence of personality disorders in the community: a global systematic review and meta-analysis. *British Journal of Psychiatry*, 216, 69–78.

World Health Organisation (1992). *ICD-10 Classification of Mental and Behavioural Disorders: Clinical Descriptions and Diagnostic Guidelines (CDDG)*. WHO: Geneva.

World Health Organisation (2024). *Clinical Descriptions and Diagnostic Requirements for ICD-11 Mental, Behavioural and Neurodevelopmental Disorders*. WHO: Geneva.

Yang M, Tyrer H, Johnson T, & Tyrer P (2022). Personality change in the Nottingham Study of Neurotic Disorder: 30 year cohort study. *Australian and New Zealand Journal of Psychiatry*, 56, 260–269.

Chapter 3

Domains of personality

Readers may be puzzled why there has been no mention in the previous chapters of some of the best known words attached to personality disorder. Why have we not come across the adjectives 'antisocial' and 'psychopathic', nor any reference to Donald Trump's famous fictional character, Hannibal Lecter, the antihero of Thomas Harris's book *The Silence of the Lambs*. And where is 'narcissistic', that sibilant polysyllable with a hint of menace, and passive aggressive personality, first used to describe non-paying patients of psychoanalysts?

The answer is that the same elements of the categories of ICD-10 personality disorder that were abolished in ICD-11 have come back in a different form as trait domains. But they are fewer and no longer dominant. Trait domains are not diagnostic categories; they are officially called qualifiers as they add flesh to the bones of the severity classification but do not stand alone.

One of the main problems with former classifications of personality disorder is that they were hijacked by celebrity. Everybody loves a good story about a memorable person, even if this bears little resemblance to the thousands of other lesser-known people who are real representations of the population. So we can all sit back as in a cinema and watch the standard-bearers of personality disorder—Hannibal Lecter talking in measured prose about cannibalism, Mrs Bennet in *Pride and Prejudice* demonstrating why no-one has any respect for her nerves, Diogenes choosing the simple life of living in a barrel, and Vincent van Gogh, having nothing better to do, chopping off his ear. These people have nothing to do with the rest of us; they have become fictionalised and a part of folklore. We relegate them to the backwoods of clinical practice, both as ordinary people and clinicians (who hardly ever used these categories in diagnostic practice), and only bring them out when we want to attack opponents, usually politicians at election time, and then forget about them.

But they are important in the context of this book as in the strategy of adaptation, they have a strong influence. It is through knowledge of

DOI: 10.4324/9781003560630-3

domains that we fashion solutions that follow the essential tone of the personality structure in a harmonious way. But to avoid getting too lyrical about them. this is how they are described in the bald language of ICD-11.

Box 3.1   Definition of trait domains (World Health Organisation, 2024, p. 559)

Trait domain specifiers may be applied to personality disorders or personality difficulty to describe the characteristics of the individual's personality that are most prominent and that contribute to personality disturbance.

Trait domains are continuous with normal personality characteristics in individuals who do not have personality disorder or personality difficulty. They are not diagnostic categories but rather represent a set of dimensions that correspond to the underlying structure of personality.

As many trait domain specifiers may be applied as necessary to describe personality functioning. Individuals with more severe personality disturbance tend to have a greater number of prominent trait domains. However, a person may have a severe personality disorder and manifest only one prominent trait domain (e.g. detachment).

(WHO, 2024, p. 559)

History of domain traits in personality

The key figure in the development of trait psychology is Gordon Allport, a psychologist from Indiana, USA. Gordon Allport rejected the psychoanalytical theories of Sigmund Freud about personality—he had a meeting with Sigmund in Vienna at the age of 22; this annoyed him as Sigmund implied he had unconscious conflicts—and developed a hard-nosed rigorous theory of personality based as much as possible on evidence. He redefined the definition of a trait, which had been used so vaguely to describe virtually every facet of human existence it had lost all credibility. He first developed, with his brother Henry, a proper classification of traits with clear definitions (Allport & Allport, 1921). He developed this further, maintaining that the true and persisting units of personality were well-defined traits, described as a hierarchy of characteristics, some more important than others, that remained constant and could be applied across a wide range of situations, so they became generalised. He first identified many individual personality features—over 4,000 of them—and then classified them into different groups. The ones that were most dominant were called cardinal traits; the ones that were most often used to describe people, such as deceitful, reserved, friendly, and suspicious, were called central traits; and those that were only manifest in certain settings, such as getting nervous when addressing a roomful of people, were labelled secondary traits (Allport, 1927). In order to satisfy the definition of a trait, the characteristic had to be persistent and consistent, particularly if it was a higher-order cardinal or central trait, and needed to have a clear definition so it did not overlap with others. Simple descriptions of behaviour (e.g., he lost his temper and tried to assault somebody) did not count as traits if they were not supported by subjective factors (e.g., he gets annoyed very easily, and you have to be very careful in your dealings with him).

But although Allport defined traits as units of personality, he did not say they constituted personality itself; they only served as a guide. This was an important message to stress. He defined personality as a 'dynamic organisation' of all the 'psychophysical systems that determine unique adjustments to the environment'. Traits were just part of the 'psychophysical systems', best regarded as building blocks. You will also note his emphasis on the environment as the substrate on which the personality needed to be adjusted.

Much later, Allport's key traits were incorporated into five patterns of thought, feeling, and behaviour that were deemed to be relatively enduring across an individual's life span. This has become known as the five-factor model, so frequently described it is usually abbreviated to FFM.

The five-factor model was developed in the 1980s by Paul Costa and Robert McCrea (McCrae & Costa, 1984; Costa & McCrae, 1992) and touted as an alternative to the classification of personality disorders in Axis II of classification, Axis I being confined to mental disorders. The FFM has now become the dominant system of normal personality classification, but its hold is precarious, and it may not last.

The characteristics of the five factors are assessed by a scoring system that allocates high scores to prominent exhibition of the trait and a low score to its absence. Here are the five factors:

Neuroticism, scoring low for those who are calm, even tempered, generally satisfied with life, and unemotional and high if they are generally anxious, temperamental, self-absorbed and self-pitying, emotional, and vulnerable.

Extraversion, scoring low for those who are reserved, isolated, quiet, passive, unemotional, and unfeeling and high for those who are affectionate, engaging, talkative, generally active, fun loving, and passionate.

Openness to experience, scoring low for those who are down to earth, uncreative, conventional, dominated by routine, incurious, and conservative and high for those who are imaginative, creative, original in thought and action, keen on variety, curious, and liberal.

Agreeableness, scoring low for those who are ruthless, suspicious, stingy and mean minded, antagonistic, hypercritical, and irritable and high for those who are soft hearted, trusting, generous, accommodating, lenient, and good natured.

Conscientiousness, scoring high for those who are self-sufficient, well ordered, and dutiful with strong commitment, and low for laziness, disorganised actions, poor interest and application, and lack of commitment.

There is no universal agreement over the big five (FFM), but they have been generated by a large number of assessments, mainly factor analyses, that have determined the associations of large numbers of traits using methods that went far beyond what Gordon Allport was able to do. Where I depart from the general approach in the five-factor model is the assumption that each factor is bipolar (i.e., that the low scores are automatically opposite to the high ones). I have come across many people in my work who are disorganised and lack self-sufficiency but when given appropriate support can be highly committed and effective.

The task force of the fifth revision of the *Diagnostic and Statistical Manual of Mental Disorders* (DSM-5) took account of many of the elements of the big five in deciding which traits they would include in their classification. Their classification was turned down by the American Psychiatric Association as it was regarded as too cumbersome and complicated, but it has managed to reform itself somewhat and make another appearance on the international stage, now as the Alternative Model of Personality Disorders (AMPD). In this classification, there are five main domains and 32 trait facets (equivalent to Allport's cardinal and central traits) (Table 3.1).

The pathological personality traits are organised into five trait domains (negative affectivity, detachment, antagonism, disinhibition, and psychoticism) and the 32 trait facets underlying them (Table 3.1) (Krueger & Hobbs, 2020). They make sense at one level, but there are major differences that differentiate them from the ICD-11 classifications. Firstly, ICD-11 did not go beyond the main trait domains, probably wisely, as the DSM trait facets have not proved particularly helpful. Secondly, the domain trait of psychoticism is not in ICD-11 as the disorder that DSM calls schizotypal disorder is regarded as part of the schizophrenia spectrum in the ICD classification and is diagnosed as schizotypy. As you might expect, I regard the ICD-11 decision as the more rational one as the features of schizotypal personality disorder are difficult to integrate with the notion of stable long-term traits that have a major influence on personality.

The third problem, and it is quite a serious one, is that the AMPD includes disinhibition and obsessionality on the same bipolar spectrum,

Table 3.1 Main domain traits and trait facets in the Alternative Model for Personality Disorders

Main trait domain	Associated facets
Negative affectivity	Anxiousness*
	Depressivity
	Emotional lability*
	Separation insecurity*
	Submissiveness
Detachment	Intimacy avoidance*
	Restricted affectivity
	Suspiciousness
	Withdrawal*
	Anhedonia*
Antagonism	Callousness
	Deceitfulness*
	Grandiosity*
	Hostility
	Manipulativeness*
Disinhibition	Attention seeking
	Distractibility*
	Impulsivity*
	Irresponsibility*
	Risk taking
	Perseveration
	Rigid perfectionism
Psychoticism	Unusual beliefs and experiences*
	Eccentricity*
	Cognitive perceptual dysregulation*

Notes: * indicates main (central) trait facet

which explains why part of Table 3.1 looks odd. Rigid perfectionism has nothing to do with distractibility; it is at the opposite pole. The problem with this is a highly personal one for me. I have assessed myself, and my conclusion, backed up by members of my family, is that I have both impulsive and obsessional personality traits in almost equal measure. According to the AMPD classification system, I cannot be on more than one point on the disinhibition scale, but I manifestly am, so the classification must be in error.

At this point, I am leaving the DSM classification as it is peripheral to the rest of this book. But I do hope that in the course of further development, this anomaly will be corrected.

The ICD-11 trait domains (or domain traits, if you prefer)

The summary description of trait domains on p. 40 includes three elements that are new to the ICD system: (a) in describing 'they are continuous with normal personality characteristics', it is emphasised they are present to some extent in everybody; (b) they give permission for disturbance in several domains to co-exist, usually in more severe personality disorders; and (c) they confirm, if confirmation was needed for those who still hanker after personality categories, that domain traits help in diagnosis by show-ing how they contribute to pathology without necessarily constituting the central part of the disorder. When people ask, 'Where are the categories of personality disorder?' the answer is a simple one: 'The categories have been subsumed into domains and are no longer diagnoses, but they are valuable qualifiers of the severity of personality disorder'.

One of the great advantages of this decision is that several trait domains may contribute simultaneously to the severity of personality disturbance without the need to change the diagnosis in any way because this is deter-mined by severity alone. Almost all investigators have found that when a large number of trait domains are regarded as pathological, the severity of the personality disorder is either moderate or severe (Tyrer & Johnson, 1996). While one of my colleagues boasted that he had just seen a patient with nine different personality disorders in the past, he can now only refer to one.

There are five trait domains in ICD-11, and these overlap considerably with the AMPD model, but they are not exactly the same, and each needs describing in detail. The domain that is missing is dependence. It can be assessed separately (Tyrer et al., 2004) and seems to be different from the others. It demands further enquiry.

The domain of negative affectivity

This name is a bit of a mouthful and has been generated by American research on the subject. One of the curious facets of American English is that it rightly shortens many of the more complex words, especially the old spelling, when these words cross the Atlantic, but then compensate for this by adding new polysyllables to words that do not need them. I still do not know what depressivity is, unless it is a word to make you feel depressed. Affect is the long-standing name for mood or emotion, and negative affec-tivity covers a range of moods that none of us would like to have if we could avoid them.

In psychiatric language between 1800 and 1980, negative affectivity was termed 'neuroticism', and the people who demonstrated neuroticism were given the label of 'neurotic'. We have dropped 'neurotic' officially, but it does not die easily, and everyone knows what is meant when, in discussion, the term 'a bit neurotic' is dropped into the conversation. It covers a panoply of attributes—the tendency to be anxious and depressed, to be hypochondriacal and always complaining, to be a constant worrier, to look on the world as a place of gloom, to mistrust others and expect the worst from them, to be prone to dependence on others, and to get irritable and angry easily. In Japan it is called *shinkeishitsu*, a personality type dominated by anxiety, sensitivity, and emotional instability that is very similar to the general neurotic syndrome described in a later chapter (Matsumoto et al., 2024).

Negative affectivity makes neuroticism a little more respectable, but it has not really changed. What has happened is that the central core of neuroticism has been added to by a range of other beliefs and feelings rather than basic emotions, which made it a bigger domain that it really is. These include symptoms that are most commonly described as borderline or emotional instability. These include suicidal feelings and actions, very poor self-perception and uncertainty, impulsive behaviours with negative consequences, feelings of utter emptiness and uselessness, and even brief psychotic episodes when the person seems to lose control and dissociate into craziness.

The question we have to ask, and this is important for lay people as well as professionals to answer, is 'Are these symptoms/feelings/episodes/ actions part of personality, or are they part of mental illness?' I have to state my position clearly. These are real and serious, often gut-wrenching problems that account for most of help-seeking behaviour in psychiatry because they create so much suffering, but they are the stuff of mental illness, not personality disorder. Personality trait domains are long-standing features that have developed in people as adaptive features at different times in human development and can be dealt with by reinforcing adaptive behaviour using nidotherapy or common-sense actions.

In the many descriptions of negative affectivity, there are elements of the description of borderline personality that complicate understanding, so I have placed them in a different place in Table 3.2.

The summary of the domain in the World Health Organisation book on ICD-11—*Clinical Descriptions and Diagnostic Requirements*—is not

Table 3.2 Differences between negative affectivity and emotional dysregulation

Negative affectivity	Borderline (emotional dysregulation) features
anxiousness	loss of emotional control
depression prone	sudden changes in mood
marked worrying	catastrophising events
poor self-esteem	self-loathing
dependence on others	fear of abandonment
gloom over future	suicidality
relative mood constancy	strong mood inconstancy
maintenance of identity	tendency to dissociation
passive acceptance	angry antagonism

reproduced here because it includes elements of emotional instability that go beyond the personality trait and should be regarded as separate for reasons that are given in the next chapter.

The core feature of negative affectivity is a constant preoccupation with many aspects of mood. Constant worry is almost a universal feature, sometimes best manifest, I think accurately, when a sufferer says, 'I'm really very worried now because there's nothing to worry about'. In such worriers, if all personal worries seem to be taken away, they have to be transferred to other members of a household. Again, the refrain often is, 'If I don't worry about it, nobody else will', and this may tend to happen in practice when families do tend to pass on all worries to one person, knowing that they can be relieved of responsibility.

Unlike the ups and downs of people with emotional deregulation, the people with high negative affectivity—and the same applies in Japan with *shinkeishitsu*—are not going from crisis to crisis but living rather restricted lives where their patterns of existence change relatively little as all change is viewed with foreboding. Their high level of anxiety had advantages in the past during dangerous phases of evolutionary development, but in modern society, it appears to have little purpose. Because their lives are restricted, self-confidence is low, and such people tend to become dependent on others and have low self-esteem.

Negative affectivity often is found in combination with other trait domains, and when it is combined with detachment or dissociality, it can lead to irritability, anger, and a high degree of suspicion of others, and these add to the anxiety even though they are not part of the anxious domain. During the preliminary discussions about ICD-11, there was a suggestion that bitterness could be given a separate category in the classification because in some people this characteristic becomes an almost dominant feature. After review, it was felt that embitterment was better thought of as an obsessive compulsive symptom.

When the personality is dominated by negative affectivity, it is almost synonymous with the person. When Jane Austen in *Pride and Prejudice* describes Mrs Bennet, it is easy to think of her as a comical figure, a frankly ludicrous player at the edge of the main plots in the novel about the romances of her daughters. Mrs Bennet lives on her nerves. Her nerves are Mrs Bennet. When she asks her husband, 'Have you no consideration for my poor nerves?' and he replies, 'You mistake me, my dear. I have the utmost respect for your nerves. They've been my constant companion these twenty years', he is expressing what he sees as the epitome of negative affectivity: an anxious, vulnerable, verbally extravagant tinder-box of ferment who finds trouble around every corner and suffers as a consequence. But, to go back to the evolutionary value of this trait, her behaviour is not unreasonable. To preserve the Bennet line, she needs her daughters to be producing children in respectable households followed by sound upbringing, and much of her anxious yabbering is devoted to this aim. It is she who is the driving force in the Bennet household, not Mr Bennet, who retires to the library when his wife takes centre stage.

Detached domain

The detached domain is at the opposite pole of negative affectivity. Emotions are kept away, and all behaviour is well-controlled. The two core features of the detachment trait domain in ICD-11 are 'the tendency to maintain interpersonal distance (social detachment) and emotional distance (emotional detachment)'. These are described separately in ICD-11:

Social detachment

Social detachment is characterised by avoidance of social interactions, lack of friendships, and avoidance of intimacy. Individuals with prominent detachment do not enjoy social interactions and avoid all kinds of social contact and social situations as far as possible. They engage in little or no 'small talk', even if initiated by others (e.g., at store check-out counters), seek out employment that does not involve interactions with others, and even refuse promotions if these would entail more interaction with others. They have few to no friends or even casual acquaintances. Their interactions with family members tend to be minimal and superficial. They rarely, if ever, engage in any intimate relationships and are not particularly interested in sexual relations.

Emotional detachment

Emotional detachment is characterised by reserve, aloofness, and limited emotional expression and experience. Individuals with prominent detachment keep to themselves as far as possible, even in obligatory social situations. They are typically aloof, responding to direct attempts at social engagement only briefly and in ways that discourage further conversation. Emotional detachment also encompasses emotional inexpressiveness, both verbally and non-verbally. Individuals with prominent detachment do not talk about their feelings, and it is difficult to discern what they might be feeling from their behaviours. In extreme cases, there is a lack of emotional experience itself, and they are non-reactive to either negative or positive events, with a limited capacity for enjoyment (World Health Organisation, 2024).

The single, not complimentary, word to describe detached individuals is cold. But there are positive aspects not in the definition. A person with a strong detached component of personality is normally an independent individual who does not wish for advice and does not take kindly to it—indeed, he or she may be very robust in rejecting it as an unnecessary and impertinent invasion into something that is intensely personal. 'Tread carefully, for you tread on my dreams', wrote Yeats, and for those who are of this bent, the treading has to be very soft indeed. So in assessing this domain, any therapist wishing to effect change has to be careful not to deviate too much from the clear aims suggested by the subject. These are likely to be very specific and precise, and changing them sometimes feels as pointless as chipping at concrete with a teaspoon.

The reason so few people receive this diagnosis, formally defined as schizoid personality disorder in ICD-10—only 0.3% received this diagnosis among all the patients diagnosed with personality disorder in the last service where I worked—is that they rarely seek advice. They comprise a very large proportion of the population that we classify as Type R, or treatment-resisting, personality disorders (Tyrer et al., 2003) as they do you not see the need for change. Often this belief is justified; many score highly on independence and commitment when it comes to personality strengths, and any suggestion that their personality might need to be changed is greeted with derision. In a later chapter, we can see the importance of adaptation in adjusting to any of the problems created by this trait domain.

The typical detached personality prefers his or her own company to that of others, is often uncomfortable in groups of people (the expression often used is an inability to 'read them'), likes tasks which can be done alone, and when interactions with others are necessary, the preference is for them to be following rules (e.g., games like chess or quizzes), rather than the uncertainty of spontaneous gatherings. None of these in themselves have any connection with autism, but in recent years, everyone seems able to find them and wish to extend this personality variation into a diagnosis of autistic spectrum disorder.

One unlikely claim is that our society is generating autism through the embrace of technology. One in 60 people now have the disorder, compared with one in 150 in 2000. Is this due to better diagnosis, more generous requirements in making the diagnosis, or a serious deficiency in our lifestyle that promotes autism? This is examined in more detail in Chapter 10, but as an illustration, it is worth looking at what is now a redundant diagnosis, Asperger's syndrome, a condition considered so important it was, until recently, a disorder that could merit a pension for life if it was formally diagnosed in Sweden.

In ICD-10, Asperger's syndrome was defined as a condition similar to autism, 'characterised by the same type of qualitative abnormalities of reciprocal social interaction that typify autism, together with a restricted, stereotyped, repetitive repertoire of interests and activities'. But there were important differences between the syndrome and autism; in particular, it was 'not associated with retardation in language or cognitive development'. In making the diagnosis, a series of other points were emphasised:

> [S]ingle words should have developed by two years of age or earlier, and that communicative phrases be used by three years of age or earlier. Self-help skills, adaptive behaviour and curiosity about the environment during the first three years should be at a level consistent with normal intellectual development. However, motor milestones may be somewhat delayed and motor clumsiness is usual (although not a necessary diagnostic feature). Isolated special skills, often related to abnormal preoccupations, are common but are not required for diagnosis. The individual exhibits and unusually intense circumscribed interest or restricted, repetitive and stereotyped pattern of behaviour, interests and activities. However it will be less usual for those to include either motor mannerisms or preoccupation with part-objects or non-functional elements of play materials.
>
> (World Health Organisation, 2024)

The description goes on:

> [T]here is a lack of any clinically significant general delay in language or cognitive development. Diagnosis requires that single words should have developed by 2 years of age or earlies and that communicative phrases be used by 3 years of age or earlier. Self-help skills, adaptive behavior, and curiosity about the environment during the first 3 years should be at a level consistent with normal intellectual development. However, motor milestones may be somewhat delayed and motor clumsiness is usual (although not necessary diagnostic feature). Isolated special skills, often related to abnormal preoccupations, are common, but are not required for diagnosis.
>
> (World Health Organisation, 2024)

How does this differ from a detached personality? Khouzam et al. (2004) explain, 'Asperger's disorder differs from adulthood schizoid personality disorder by the predominance of stereotyped behavior and interests that severely impair social interactions', but when you look at the main criteria for diagnosis—'restricted, stereotyped, repetitive repertoire of interests and activities'—this is no different from a forester working alone in a woodland where he has to thin out all trees that are close together as these are more likely to be blown over in storms. If he likes the job, prefers working alone, and wants to continue it, should this really be described as a 'restricted, stereotyped, repetitive repertoire'?

No, the diagnosis of Asperger's syndrome was rightly removed in ICD–11. If you read the description of the syndrome again, it seems only to be a combination of clumsiness, focused unusual interests, and repetition of these that constitute the diagnosis; all the other features are negative ones that differentiate it from classical autism. Steve Silberman (2015), in his rip-roaring optimistic book *Neurotribes,* is right to praise diversity here rather than give all these people a pathology, adding 'not all the features of atypical human operating systems are bugs' (Wing, 1981).

Disinhibited domain

Disinhibition links together an old quotation adapted from J.M. Barrie's *Peter Pan.* 'Doing what you like is freedom; liking what you do is happiness'. Those who are disinhibited see happiness and freedom beckoning to them continually, and it does not need much for action to follow, but it often does not go in the direction in which it points. When we put it into the language of ICD-11, we can see its hazards:

> The core feature of the disinhibition trait domain is the tendency to act rashly based on immediate external or internal stimuli (i.e. sensations, emotions, thoughts), without consideration of potential negative consequences.

The definition goes on to include four inter-related elements:

Impulsivity

Individuals with prominent disinhibition tend to act rashly based on whatever is compelling at the moment, without consideration of negative consequences for themselves or others, including putting themselves or others at physical risk. They have difficulty delaying reward or satisfaction and tend to pursue immediately available short-term pleasures or potential benefits. In this way, the trait is strongly associated with such behaviours as substance use, gambling, and impulsive sexual activity.

Distractibility

Individuals with prominent disinhibition also have difficulty staying focused on important and necessary tasks that require sustained effort.

They quickly become bored or frustrated with difficult, routine, or tedious tasks and are easily distracted by extraneous stimuli, such as others' conversations. Even in the absence of distractions, they have difficulty keeping their attention focused and persisting on tasks and tend to scan the environment for more enjoyable options.

Irresponsibility

Individuals with prominent disinhibition are unreliable and lack a sense of accountability for their actions. As a result, they often do not complete work assignments or perform expected duties; they fail to meet deadlines, do not follow through on commitments and promises, and are late to or miss formal and informal appointments and meetings because they allow themselves to become engaged in something more compelling that has caught their attention.

Recklessness

Individuals with prominent disinhibition lack an appropriate sense of caution. They tend to overestimate their abilities and thus frequently do things that are beyond their skill level, without considering potential safety risks. 'Individuals with prominent disinhibition may engage in reckless driving or dangerous sports or perform other activities that put them or others in physical danger without sufficient preparation or training' (World Health Organisation, 2024, p. 562).

Many of the consequences of disinhibition are classified separately as mental disorders. Alcoholism, substance misuse, sexual addiction, attention deficit-hyperactivity disorder (ADHD), and a new disorder in ICD-11, gaming disorder, can all be consequences of disinhibition, but because they are such prominent conditions in their own right, the role of the underlying trait domain is often forgotten. Fyodor Dostoevsky understood the role of disinhibition when he wrote *The Gambler* in 1866.

First, the recklessness:

'But gamblers know how a man can sit for almost twenty-four hours at cards, without looking to right, or to left'. 'Can I possibly not understand myself that I'm a lost man? But—why can't I resurrect? Yes! it only takes being calculating and patient at least once in your life and—that's all'.

Next, the 'immediately available short-term pleasures':

No, it was not the money that I valued—what I wanted was to make all this mob of Heintzes, hotel proprietors, and fine ladies of Baden talk about me, recount my story, wonder at me, extol my doings, and worship my winnings.

Finally, the irresponsible difficulty in 'keeping attention focused and persisting on tasks' when there is an immediate bonus right in front of you:

> Well, what, what new thing can they say to me that I don't know myself? And is that the point? The point here is that—one turn of the wheel, and everything changes, and these same moralizers will be the first (I'm sure of it) to come with friendly jokes to congratulate me. And they won't all turn away from me as they do now. Spit on them all! What am I now? *Zéro*. What may I be tomorrow? Tomorrow I may rise from the dead and begin to live anew! I may find the man in me before he's lost!

In the same way in which detachment is sometimes mis-identified as disinhibition is mis-identified as ADHD, particularly when diagnosed in adult life. The two main diagnostic features needed to make a diagnosis of ADHD at any age are inattention and the combination of hyperactivity and impulsiveness.

The features in the hyperactivity-impulsivity section include 'excessive motor activity', 'having difficulty sitting still', 'physical restlessness and a sense of discomfort when sitting still', and 'having a tendency to act in response to immediate stimuli without deliberation or consideration of risks and consequences (e.g. engaging in behaviours with potential for physical injury; impulsive decisions; reckless driving)'.

The wording 'having a tendency' is much more than a nod to the disinhibited domain; it is a prominent signpost. At the very least, a diagnosis of personality difficulty or mild personality disorder with prominent disinhibition features should be considered in those with ADHD.

Dissocial domain

The dissocial domain is given considerable attention in ICD-11, and its full description is illuminating as it highlights two of its central features (Box 3.2).

Box 3.2.   Characteristics of the dissocial trait domain (World Health Organisation, 2024, pp. 561–562

The core feature of the dissociality trait domain is disregard for the rights and feelings of others, encompassing both self-centredness and lack of empathy. Common manifestations of dissociality, not all of which may be present in a given individual at a given time, include the following:

Self-centredness

Self-centredness in individuals with prominent dissociality is manifested in a sense of entitlement, believing and acting as if they deserve—without further justification—whatever they want, preferentially above what others may want or need, and that this 'fact' should be obvious to others. Self-centredness can be manifested both actively/intentionally and passively/unintentionally. Active—and usually intentional—manifestations of self-centredness include expectation of others' admiration, attention-seeking behaviours to ensure being the centre of others' focus, and negative behaviours (e.g. anger, 'temper tantrums', denigrating others) when the admiration and attention that the individual expects are not granted. Typically, such individuals believe that they have many admirable qualities, that their accomplishments are outstanding, that they have achieved or will achieve greatness, and that others should admire them. Passive and unintentional manifestations of self-centredness reflect a kind of obliviousness that other individuals matter as much as oneself. In this aspect of dissociality, the individual's concern is with their own needs, desires and comfort, and those of others simply are not considered.

Lack of empathy

Lack of empathy is manifested in indifference to whether one's actions inconvenience others or hurt them in any way (e.g. emotionally, socially, financially, physically). As a result, individuals with prominent dissociality are often deceptive and manipulative, exploiting people and situations to get what they want and think they deserve. This may include being mean and physically aggressive. In the extreme, this aspect of dissociality can be manifested in callousness with regard to others' suffering and ruthlessness in obtaining one's goals, such that these individuals may be physically violent with little to no provocation, and may even take pleasure in inflicting pain and harm. Note that this aspect of dissociality does not necessarily imply that individuals with prominent dissociality do not cognitively understand the feelings of others; rather, they are not concerned about them and instead are likely to use this understanding to exploit others.

These two features, self-centeredness and lack of empathy, cannot help but draw attention to the related term 'psychopathy'.

ICD-11 has disregarded 'psychopathy' entirely in its descriptive and diagnostic guidelines. When our revision group looked at the criteria for the dissociality domain, there was so much overlap between these and those for psychopathy that we could not find any justification for a separate description. But psychopathy is a word that has stuck very firmly in people's minds and cannot be ignored. It has a colourful history in which it is often difficult to separate the science from the fantasy, especially as the fantasy makes for much better reading—it is almost impossible to ignore it in crime novels. But here, I am going to stick to the science but add a little to lighten the load.

The term only became popular in the late 19th century when the German psychiatrist Julius Koch attempted a classification of mental disorders that (fortunately) did not catch on at first, as in his three books he described all mental illness as either hereditary or acquired psychopathic inferiorities (*Die psychopathischen Minderwertigkeiten*). Criminals were just one group within this broad canvas, but for some reason that I cannot fathom, they became particularly attached to antisocial behaviour. Much later, this was taken up by Hervey Cleckley, a psychiatrist from Augusta in Georgia (who was also educated in England), who wrote a popular book, *The Mask of Sanity*, in 1941, which also delineated the key features of psychopathy from his clinical experience.

His descriptions were brilliant: hence, the success of his book and the adoption of many of the terms he used. According to Cleckley, the true psychopath was glib and universally charming, had no sense of any personal responsibility, was a pathological and persuasive liar, took no responsibility for their actions no matter how they turned out, lacked any remorse, had no long-term goals, was grossly egocentric and grandiose, lacked empathy, and was sexually promiscuous. He also stated that their lives always ended in failure, but, please note, he was only seeing the unsuccessful ones in correctional institutions.

There are many who have these qualities, at least to some extent, who have no criminal convictions and are highly successful. There is even one, Donald Trump, who has a criminal conviction which seems to have made him even more successful. The problem with the term 'psychopathy' is the same problem we have with 'borderline'; it covers a large number of people and so lacks specificity. At one extreme, we have the characters beloved by filmmakers (Who can ever forget *Psycho*? Alfred Hitchcock only needed the first two syllables) and novelists (Thomas Harris, author of *Silence of the Lambs*, who invented Hannibal Lecter but insisted 'I don't think I ever made up anything'), and, at the other extreme, we have highly successful business executives and entrepreneurs who seem to have identical qualities. What is the use of a term that can include all these people?

But psychopathy has certainly not disappeared in forensic psychiatry. This is largely due to Robert Hare, whose core publication, 'The Psychopathy Checklist' (revised version PCR-R, published in 2003) is the key measure now used to identify psychopathy.

'The Psychopathy Checklist' rates individuals on 30 items the cover lack of empathy and guilt, phone emotions, the manipulation of others, the grandiose sense of self-worth, failure to take care of obligations, exploiting others again, and showing strong evidence of antisocial behaviour starting in early childhood. Hare essentially formalised Hervey Cleckley's descriptions into operational criteria for psychopathy and has been followed consistently by forensic services across the globe. But the PCL-R, despite being a core measure for psychopathy, has not been free of controversy, mainly because its items combine past criminal behaviour and personality disorder in a way that many experts feel is unjustified (Blackburn, 2005; Cooke et al., 2007). In the Dangerous and Severe Personality Disorder Programme, discussed later in this book, a score of 30 on the PCL-R was said to be diagnostic of psychopathy, but in many cases, most of the score was made up of historical criminal acts that were very different from current personality function (Tyrer et al., 2004) and had also shifted over time. Our experience, reinforced by other discussions (with Essi Viding), supported our conclusion that psychopathy should be left out of the ICD-11 classification.

The other key authority on psychopathy was David Henderson, a celebrated Scottish psychiatrist who studied under Adolf Meyer at Johns Hopkins Hospital and who had a close interest in the clinical outcomes of his patients. Based on this experience alone—always a useful first step in research but never a definitive one—he defined three groups of psychopaths and published a book after a series of lectures, *Psychopathic States* (Henderson, 1939). He described three types of psychopaths. The first was very similar to that of criminal psychopathy and was self-centred, selfish, callous, aggressive, and dangerous. The second was the inadequate psychopath, a person who lived off society by swindling and cheating, was frequently in prison for minor offences but who was not violent, and the third group, the most controversial, being eccentric people who went against social norms. He included individuals such as Lawrence of Arabia in this group, but now, most would consider these to be on the detached spectrum and not necessarily regarded as disordered.

Henderson's contribution to the subject was considerable. His wish for psychopathy to be taken seriously as a psychiatric disorder led to the opening of the first hospital in the country to treat this condition in the form of a therapeutic community. This was named the Henderson Hospital, and it closed in 2008 after an interesting 64-year history, during which it was often in the headlines.

Anankastic domain

The ICD-11 describes the core feature of the anankastia trait domain as 'a narrow focus on one's rigid standard of perfection and of right and wrong, on controlling one's own and others' behaviour, and on controlling situations to ensure conformity to these standards'. It includes the following:

Perfectionism

Perfectionism is manifested in concern with social rules, obligations, and norms of right and wrong; scrupulous attention to detail; rigid, systematic, day-to-day routines; excessive scheduling and planning; and an emphasis on organisation, orderliness, and neatness. Individuals with prominent anankastia have a very clear and detailed personal sense of perfection and imperfection that extends beyond community standards to encompass the individual's idiosyncratic notions of what is perfect and right. They believe strongly that everyone should follow all rules exactly and meet all obligations. Individuals with prominent anankastia may redo the work of others because it does not meet their perfectionistic standards. They have difficulty in interpersonal relationships because they hold others to the same standards as themselves, and are inflexible in their views.

Emotional and behavioural constraint are also highlighted:

Emotional and behavioural constraint is manifested in rigid control over emotional expression, stubbornness and inflexibility, risk-avoidance, perseveration and deliberativeness. Individuals with prominent anankastic traits tightly control their own emotional expression, and disapprove of others' displays of emotion. They are inflexible and lack spontaneity, stubbornly insisting on following set schedules and adhering to plans. Their risk-avoidance includes both refusal to engage in obviously risky activities and a more general overconcern about avoiding potential negative consequences of any activity. They often perseverate and have difficulty disengaging from tasks because they are perceived as not yet perfect down to the last detail. They are highly deliberative and have difficulty making decisions due to concern that they have not considered every aspect and all alternatives to ensure that the right decision is made'.

There is considerable overlap between the anankastic trait and obsessive compulsive disorder (OCD), but the two conditions can be easily differentiated (Mancebo et al., 2005). The key difference is that those with the anankastic trait regard it as a positive attribute of their personality (i.e., it is ego-syntonic), whereas those with obsessive compulsive disorder are very distressed by their symptoms and want them to be removed (i.e., they are ego-dystonic). Mancebo give one example of the need to construct complicated lists of future actions:

[A] patient with OCD makes lists because they are afraid they will be responsible for something terrible happening if they do not follow their list exactly. In contrast, a person with obsessive compulsive personality disorder will justify excessive list-making with the rationale that it is a reasonable use of their time and prevents them from forgetting important tasks.

(Mancebo et al., 2005, p. 201)

It is much easier for those with the anankastic trait to defend their actions and behaviour than it is with other trait domains. Our current societal structure rewards those who are meticulous, accurate, and reliable, and so many who find this characteristic tiresome and irritating are put on the back foot.

It is not the anankastic person who has to adapt to them; it is they who have to adapt to the worthy but annoying world of the obsessional.

References

Allport FH & Allport GW (1921). Personality traits: their classification and measurement. *The Journal of Abnormal Psychology and Social Psychology*, 16, 6–40.

Allport GW (1927). Concepts of trait and personality. *Psychological Bulletin*, 24, 284–293.

Blackburn R (2005). Psychopathy as a personality construct. In: S Strack (ed.), *Handbook of Personology and Psychopathology*, pp. 271–291. John Wiley & Sons.

Cooke DJ, Michie C, & Skeem J (2007). Understanding the structure of the Psychopathy Checklist—Revised: an exploration of methodological confusion. *British Journal of Psychiatry*, (Suppl 49), s39–s50.

Costa PT & McCrae RR (1992). The five-factor model of personality and its relevance to personality disorders. *Journal of Personality Disorders*, 6, 343–359.

Dostoevsky F (2018). *The Gambler*. Read & Co Classics. (First published to pay off his gambling debts in 1866).

Hare RD (2003). *The Psychopathy Checklist—Revised* (2nd edition). Toronto: Multi-Health Systems.

Henderson DK (1939). *Psychopathic States*. New York: W.W. Norton.

Khouzam HR, El-Gabalawi F, Pirwani N, & Priest F (2004). Asperger's disorder: a review of its diagnosis and treatment. *Comprehensive Psychiatry*, 45, 184–191.

Koch J (1891–3). *Die psychopathischen Minderwertigkeiten* (3 vols.). Ravensburg: Maier.

Krueger RF & Hobbs KA (2020). An overview of the DSM-5 Alternative Model of Personality Disorders. *Psychopathology*, 53, 126–132.

Mancebo MC, Eisen JL, Grant JE, & Rasmussen SA (2005). Obsessive compulsive personality disorder and obsessive compulsive disorder: clinical characteristics, diagnostic difficulties, and treatment. *Annals of Clinical Psychiatry*, 17, 197–204.

Matsumoto H, Uchino T, Funatogawa T, Mizuno M, & Nemoto T (2024). Characteristics of patients with neurotic disorders requiring long-term treatment: relationship to "nervous personality" as described in Morita's *Shinkeishitsu* theory. *Psychiatry & Clinical Neuroscience Reports*, 3, e70039.

McCrae RR & Costa PT, Jr (1984). *Emerging Lives, Enduring Dispositions: Personality in Adulthood*. Boston, MA: Little, Brown and Co.

Silberman S (2015). *Neurotribes. The Legacy of Autism and the Future of Neurodiversity*. Random House.

Tyrer P & Johnson T (1996). Establishing the severity of personality disorder. *American Journal of Psychiatry*, 153, 1593–1597.

Tyrer P, Mitchard S, Methuen C, & Ranger M (2003). Treatment-rejecting and treatment-seeking personality disorders: Type R and Type S. *Journal of Personality Disorders*, 17, 265–270.

Tyrer P, Morgan J, & Cicchetti D (2004). The Dependent Personality Questionnaire (DPQ): a screening instrument for dependent personality. *International Journal of Social Psychiatry*, 50, 10–17.

Wing L (1981). Asperger's syndrome: a clinical account. *Psychological Medicine*, 11, 115–129.

World Health Organisation (2024). *Clinical Descriptions and Diagnostic Requirements for ICD-11 Mental, Behavioural and Neurodevelopmental Disorders*. WHO: Geneva.

Chapter 4

The borderline conundrum

It is argued elsewhere in this book that the condition commonly described as borderline personality disorder cannot possibly be regarded as a true personality disorder for many reasons. Some might disagree, but the subject certainly deserves a separate chapter. I first need to show the wording of what has been variously described as a redundant addition to classification (Mulder et al., 2020), an ensuring continuity (Bach et al., 2022), the enhancement of clinical utility (Sharan et al., 2023), and a condition that 'has no basis in the scientific study of personality and is used indiscriminately to describe myriad negative interactions in human relationships that have cause far beyond personality function, extending from simple disagreement to total functional breakdown' (Mulder & Tyrer, 2023).

This is what is known as the 'borderline pattern', sometimes called the 'borderline pattern descriptor' or 'borderline pattern specifier' in the ICD-11 classification (Box 4.1).

Box 4.1. The borderline pattern specifier in ICD-11 (World Health Organisation, 2024, p. 554)

The borderline pattern descriptor may be applied to individuals whose pattern of personality disturbance is characterised by a pervasive pattern of instability of interpersonal relationships, self-image, and affects and marked impulsivity, as indicated by many of the following: frantic efforts to avoid real or imagined abandonment; a pattern of unstable and intense interpersonal relationships; identity disturbance, manifested in markedly and persistently unstable self-image or sense of self; a tendency to act rashly in states of high negative affect, leading to potentially self-damaging behaviours; recurrent episodes of self-harm; emotional instability due to marked reactivity of

---

DOI: 10.4324/9781003560630-4

mood; chronic feelings of emptiness; inappropriate intense anger or difficulty controlling anger; and transient dissociative symptoms or psychotic-like features in situations of high affective arousal.

Now the text of this 'pattern specifier' can be analysed for the features that might make it a personality disorder or exclude it as a separate disorder. Here are the reasons for exclusion:

1 It is a list of symptoms and behaviours, not of personality traits.
2 It has never been an advantage in human evolution, unlike other domain traits.
3 It pursues a complex course that is quite unlike any other personality disorder.
4 It is better regarded as a mental illness, a condition that has been externally imposed on the person (often described as ego-dystonic) and not an accepted ingrained personality structure (ego-syntonic).
5 Its manifestations overlap with almost every other condition in mental health and therefore have very little specificity.
6 It is not a condition to which it is possible to adapt.

These points are not new; I put them forth 15 years ago (Tyrer, 2009) and have not seen anything new to change my mind. But there is a counter-argument that should be considered also. Here are six strong reasons why borderline is regarded by many as a very useful and acceptable diagnosis:

1 Most people presenting to services with personality disorder have borderline symptoms.
2 It has a well-described and easily recognisable set of features that all psychiatrists can recognise.
3 It has attracted more research interest than any other personality disorder.
4 It is the only personality disorder that has confirmed evidence-based treatments.
5 It is the personality disorder with the most impact on public mental health because of its association with suicidality.
6 It is the only personality disorder for which you can get insurance cover (in some countries).

It could be argued that these six reasons in favour and six against are finely balanced, but when scientific principles are applied in the same way Gordon

Allport examined personality traits, the points in favour of the diagnosis fade away. Some clinicians recoil from science in respect to personality—it is too delicate a subject for this type of rigorous examination—but no subject can argue it should be in a science-free zone. Let me examine each of the points in favour of the diagnosis in turn.

1 Most people presenting to services with personality disorder have borderline symptoms. Yes, indeed. I once took part in a debate with George Vaillant, an incisive and witty Harvard professor, well known in the field of psychology. Fortunately, I was on the same side as George in a debate about the value of borderline personality disorder. Yes, indeed, George said, borderline was a very popular diagnosis. 'At Harvard 70% of the patients we see are borderline. I have a suggestion to make; let's regard all the patients as borderline until proved otherwise'. This shows the compass of the diagnosis is so broad that it almost excludes, or joins up with, almost all other mental disorders. A good diagnosis has to be both highly sensitive and specific; in other words, it identifies all the likely cases of the condition, and the ones it does identify are all accurate and fit the requirements of the diagnosis. Borderline personality disorder is extremely sensitive as a diagnosis—it can be attributed to almost anybody who loses their temper in an argument and storms out of a room—but it is extraordinarily non-specific as it is so difficult to determine what exactly is the core of the personality behind the disorder.

2 'It has a well-described and easily recognisable set of features that all psychiatrists can recognise'. This is true—it explains why so many clinicians say out loud, 'That's a typical borderline' when they hear a case description. But the individual elements do not join together. In the rather dry language of personality psychology, this is illustrated by Krueger and Hobbs:

> This leaves other characteristics (beyond those that form the understandable foci of borderline PD intervention) relatively less well conceptualized from an intervention angle. For example, emotional lability (a key criterion B facet) combined with risk taking (a separate criterion B facet that tends to vary relatively independently of emotional lability) is a different presentation from emotional lability combined with rigid perfectionism (a third criterion B facet). What is needed are case conceptualization flow charts linked to the multidimensional nature of PD variation. Reducing dimensional information to singular labels (e.g., 'high on detachment') may be as problematic for reliability and case conceptualization as classical PD labels.
>
> (Krueger & Hobbs, 2020, p. 130)

Borderline borders on all traits but does not belong to any condition, summarised by Akiskal and his colleagues as a floating adjective in search of a noun (Akiskal et al., 1985).

3 'It has attracted more research interest than any other personality disorder'. This is also true, but research interest is also related to puzzlement and uncertainty. The more a subject confuses, the more it needs to be studied to resolve the confusion. It does not make the diagnosis more valid.

4 'It is the only personality disorder that has confirmed evidence-based treatments'. This is a very strong point in favour of the continued use of the term. But, as George Vaillant pointed out, there are so many people who seek treatment for personality problems who seem to fit into the diagnosis, so it explains the literature. The contrary argument that a better, more precise diagnosis would lead to better more precise treatments has not been tested.

5 'It is the personality disorder with the most impact on public mental health because of its association with suicidality'. There is little doubt that suicide prevention, no matter how elusive, is a public health issue, but it is already a key part of treatment for other conditions, notably depressive disorder, and a new diagnosis, non-suicidal self-injury (NSSI), is being recognised without the need for the borderline diagnostic tag.

6 'It is the only personality disorder for which you can get insurance cover (in some countries)'. This is not a good reason for a diagnosis. But I could understand the concern of a red-faced man in the audience of a talk I was giving on ICD-11 personality disorder. I noticed he was getting increasingly agitated, and at the end of the talk, he expostulated, 'You cannot remove the diagnosis of borderline—it is not possible—we need it for the purpose of insurance, don't you understand?' He was the chief representative of a German insurance company. I could only reply that the insurance industry should not be the arbiter of diagnosis in psychiatry.

When the ICD-11 revision group began its work on a new classification of personality disorder, it was very confident it had identified four of the five domain traits accurately—it was less confident about the disinhibition one—but it had serious trouble with the borderline one. When the data were examined closely, the borderline domain dipped into the territory of most of the other domains like an unwelcome visitor at a party. It was very comfortable at high tea as part of the negative affective domain, in which all the emotions have dominance; it crashed unwanted into the dissocial domain, where anger, resentment, and paranoia were having Irish coffee; jumped in unexpectedly at the impulsive domain, where there was reckless eating and drinking with new untried recipes; and even called in briefly to the anankastic parlour, where the highly organised team were still completing the planning of their evening meal.

Of course these data were published more prosaically as a scientific paper, but the message was the same as my metaphorical musings: borderline did not have a domain structure; it just invaded all the others but did not belong in any of them (Mulder et al., 2016). Although I had always been sceptical about the value of borderline as a diagnosis—in a book I edited in 1988, I suggested that if it was 'a mixture of personality and mental state abnormality it would be more appropriately described as a clinical syndrome than as a personality disorder' (Tyrer, 1988, p. 25)—my view was reinforced by all in the ICD-11 group.

The consequence of our debate in light of all these findings, the ICD-11 revision committee concluded that borderline/emotionally unstable personality disorder did not belong in the classification; it had to be excluded. It was already excluded from the main diagnostic system that recorded personality by severity only and had no defined categories, but now it could not even be regarded as one of the key domains of the personality structure.

So the most popular boy in the school was being expelled. It is not difficult to imagine the reaction. All around the world, those who were determined to retain the label of borderline personality disorder jumped into action. This included the originators of the key psychological treatments described later in this chapter, as the loss of their precious group would seem to invalidate their work; the insurance industry, which had been persuaded to provide cover for the treatment of this condition; the drug industry, which loved providing new treatments for the condition even though they were ineffective (Stoffers-Winterling et al., 2022) and sometimes led to dependence (Tyrer, 2024); and (some of) those with lived experience who had, for the first time, found an explanation for their symptoms and felt better for it (Lester et al., 2020).

To attempt to square a very round circle that the ICD-11 group had made perfectly clear should not have its shape altered—'personality dysfunction is best represented as a single dimension of severity and does not include any categories'—the World Health Organisation, under its very diligent ICD-11 coordinator, Geoffrey Reed, convened a meeting in Heidelberg, where it was agreed with the borderline defenders that the frantic attempts to avoid abandonment could be staved off. Borderline could be included: not as a diagnosis, not as a domain, but as a pattern specifier. The arguments for including this were pretty weak, but they satisfied the complainants. In the marvellous way in which the English language can be used in diplomatic code, the justification was:

This qualifier may enhance clinical utility by facilitating the identification of individuals who may respond to certain psychotherapeutic treatments. Whether it will provide information that is non-redundant with the trait domain qualifiers is an empirical question.

(Reed, 2018)

So the boy who was expelled could now come back to school. But he had to sit in a separate classroom of his own and would not mix with the other boys; he would continue visits from his admirers.

For those who are devoted to treating people with this disorder and are still convinced the diagnosis is helpful, it is necessary first to look at the published evidence of their efficacy.

Until the mid-1970s, the idea of untreatability persisted, but then a paper by Gunderson and Singer in 1975 changed perceptions markedly. This brought borderline to the top of the personality pile and gave clinicians and patients hope again. Elsewhere in this book, I have pointed out all the problems of borderline personality disorder as a diagnosis, but there is no doubt that its embrace by so many practitioners and patients has helped stimulate interest in the subject.

There are now six established or promising treatments for personality disorder. None of them is connected to nidotherapy but they are worth describing in some detail so the reader can determine to what extent they can be regarded as adaptive.

1.   Dialectical behaviour therapy

Dialectical behaviour therapy (DBT) is the treatment with most evidence in its favour. It was developed by a charismatic psychologist, Marsha Linehan, who nowadays would also be called an 'expert by experience', as she developed the treatment for the condition she experienced herself as a young woman when she was repeatedly suicidal. It is therefore not surprising that her treatment focuses mainly on the prevention of suicidal behaviour, and this is where her results have been most successful. But no study has had a large enough sample to test whether it actually reduces suicide. Only one review suggests any intervention reduces death; that was good community care practised before current managerial community care took over (Simmonds et al., 2001). As the population with borderline symptoms has a suicide rate of about 10% over time (Paris, 2003), a study to demonstrate a positive effect of treatment should not be impossible but would need a follow-up period of many years (Paris & Zweig-Frank, 2001; Jenkins et al., 2002).

The initial paper on dialectical behaviour therapy focused on severe emotional dysregulation and suicidal behaviour (Linehan et al., 1991). It was subsequently taken over by the borderline lobby, a term that is not meant to be offensive but describes a group with a common focus that is pursued diligently. I think they got it wrong. Throughout the development of DBT, Marsha Linehan has argued that her treatment is primarily focused on managing emotional dysregulation and not personality disorder. She argues that this dysregulation comes from the combination of emotional vulnerability and environments that are invalidating. An invalidating environment is one where there are 'persistent discrepancies between private experience and what others in the environment describe' (Linehan, 2015, p. 8), and this mismatch promotes emotional dysregulation. The lack of faith in the environment—mainly personal and social and often developed early in life—leads to large areas of function becoming increasingly dysregulated, and this extends right to the core of the self so that even the identity of the person is questioned. In managing this dysregulation, a broad range of strategies is used: the teaching of new skills, the adoption of mindfulness and acceptance strategies, and the promotion of new behaviours. DBT is the most frequently recommended treatment for borderline personality disorder by NICE (National Institute for Health and Care Excellence, 2009).

It is also relevant that DBT is not focused on any of the other types of personality disorder. It does not pretend to go beyond emotional instability as the main area of treatment.

2.   Mentalisation-based therapy

Mentalisation-based treatment (MBT) was specifically developed for borderline personality disorder. It differs from dialectical behaviour therapy by deriving much of its content from psychodynamic practice and attachment theory. Mentalising, its key component, is the capacity to pay attention and appreciate both our own and others' feelings, thoughts, motives, hopes, desires, and motivations. When achieved, it accentuates self-understanding and self-confidence. It is particularly lacking in borderline personality disorder, and the main effort of MBT is to improve mentalising so what Antonovsky called a 'sense of coherence' (Antonovsky, 1979) is improved, and a more stable representation of the self is presented to the world. A great deal depends on the nature of the therapeutic relationship. In several ways, MBT shares characteristics with dialectical behaviour therapy (discussed later), but it includes more individual and group psychoanalytic therapy. The core element is the somewhat elusive concept of mentalisation, the process that allows us to connect with other people in a way that makes understandable our feelings and those of others. Consequently, it is a central part of our relationships with other people (Bateman & Fonagy, 2009, 2016). It also is closely linked to attachment theory, and much attention in treatment is paid to the need to develop secure attachments, so often lacking in those with personality disorder.

Mentalisation-based treatment has been evaluated in several controlled trials and is undoubtedly effective, but it is uncertain what constitutes its key ingredients. Is it the structured format of the treatment, one that is unusual for a psychodynamic intervention; is it the training leading to the ability to mentalise; is it the special relationship with the therapist; or is it a combination of all three of these?

What is very clear is that both DBT and MBT are treatments to eliminate, neutralise, overcome, and compensate for in different ways the pathology of emotional dysregulation. They differ from nidotherapy in that they do not attempt to harness personality disturbance but to remove it. You do not adapt to emotional dysregulation; it is a damaging component of functioning, and there is no way it can be spun into a positive. Unlike the domains of personality disturbance, a fouled-up capacity to deal with emotions is not, nor has it ever been, an asset in evolutionary development.

3. Cognitive behaviour therapy

Cognitive behaviour therapy (CBT) has been an established treatment for mood and stress disorders, eating disorders, and trauma for many years. It was adapted for the management of personality disorders by its inventor, Tim Beck, and has enjoyed some success. Aaron Tim (now known mainly as Tim) Beck introduced cognitive therapy for depression in the 1960s and has written about its adaptation for all types of personality disorder for over 30 years (Beck et al., 1990, 2015).

But CBT for personality disorders is not fundamentally different from its use in other disorders. It focuses on cognitive restructuring, examining beliefs in a different way and, at its core, follows the standard CBT approach by identifying dysfunctional beliefs and discovering alternative positive ones. But the time scale of treatment is longer than in other disorders and includes education, problem-solving, behavioural experiments (e.g., testing out new strategies and recording progress with diaries), and homework. This requires application and commitment, and most people have to be well motivated to complete it successfully, so, not surprisingly, it is those with emotional instability who are most likely to be fully engaged with this form of treatment. It has been shown to be successful in both the short term and long term in reducing suicidal behaviour (Davidson et al., 2006, 2010).

It is important to record that almost all the studies in the recent past have used the old diagnostic systems for recording personality disorder, so we do not know if the treatments are best focused on mild, moderate, or severe personality disorder. One study by Bateman and Fonagy (2009) found milder forms of personality disturbance could be treated equally well by good all-round care, relabelled as structured clinical management, when compared with mentalisation-based treatment, but more severe personality disorder responded better to MBT. Follow-up after eight years showed similar outcomes, with MBT showing superiority in gainful activities (Bateman et al., 2021).

4. Transference-focused therapy

Transference-focused therapy is driven by psychoanalytical theory. It was introduced first by Otto Kernberg (2016) but developed as a treatment model with the help of Clarkin and Yeomans (Clarkin et al., 2007). It too is used for the treatment of borderline pathology and focuses on the 'unreconciled and contradictory representations of the self' that lead to disturbed relationships with others. The treatment is named as these distorted perceptions are examined in the relationship of the patient with the therapist, or transference. Attempts are made to integrate the different parts of self and object representations as these are judged to have been separated and led to distorted perceptions.

5. Schema-focused therapy

Schema-focused therapy is based on the concept that, in childhood, 'dysfunctional schemata' that prevent the secure development of identity are formed, are accentuated by trauma, and lead to negative coping strategies (Young et al., 2003). Schemas are complex patterns of thought and behaviour that go beyond dysfunctional thoughts, so treatment generally extends beyond cognitive behavioural therapy. The patient-therapist relationship is used to teach the person the essentials of a trusting relationship, known as limited reparenting.

Schema-focused therapy has had limited evaluation; the largest study was a randomised trial by Giesen-Bloo et al. (2006) that showed superiority of schema therapy over transference-focused therapy in patients with borderline personality disorder over a three-year period.

6. Cognitive analytic therapy

Cognitive analytic therapy (CAT) is an offshoot of cognitive behaviour therapy and object relations theory but has some distinct differences (Ryle, 1997, 2004). It normally consists of up to 24 individual sessions of treatment. Anthony Ryle, who developed it, was neither a psychoanalyst nor a psychologist and developed his ideas while working as a student health officer. It is often said that Leonardo da Vinci was allowed to be so original in his thinking as he had no formal education and so was not held back by the stultifying theories of his age. Anthony Ryle followed the same bent; because he worked on his own, his ideas could be brought forward without interference. He was frustrated by the formalities of psychodynamic and cognitive theory and rejected them:

> Psychoanalysis makes an attempt that is proper in range and ambition, but it has become trapped by theoretical confusion and restricted in its method by institutional pressures. Cognitive and behavioural approaches, on the other hand, offer effective therapies over a limited range on the basis of theories that attend to only segments of human experience.
>
> (Ryle et al., 2014)

I have called CAT a 'humanised and skilled psychotherapy' (Tyrer, 2013) as, like nidotherapy, it is not restricted by diagnostic boundaries and assesses every condition in mental health. At interviews, it concentrates on emphasising relationships in a broad and open way and, if they are found to get complicated, can be followed with the aid of a map that helps create a diagrammatic reformulation (Potter, 2020). CAT makes a special point of emphasising the role of 'structural dissociation' in the development of separate (reciprocal) self-states, between which patients with borderline presentation can abruptly switch when under stress. Ryle examines dissociation minutely and helps people understand its use and misuse as a coping strategy. The languages of professional practice, neuroscience, and diagnosis are not ignored in cognitive analytical therapy, but the meaning of these labels is given to the patient in context, allowing it to be a starting point for collaboration and exploration. CAT can provide a complementary alternative to a neurobiological model of mental illness. It is best summarised in a recent review that ends with a plea:

> [I]t is hoped that there will remain room in the NHS for a psychological therapy based on a relational and developmental paradigm, as an alternative to an overreliance on manualised therapies and interventions based on diagnostic clusters linked to a neurobiological understanding of mental illness.
>
> (Ryle et al., 2014, p. 266)

Although the most careful evaluation of cognitive analytical therapy, a randomised trial published by Chanen et al. (2008), showed no superiority over the control condition of 'good clinical care', those treated with CAT improved more rapidly.

7. Acceptance and commitment therapy

Acceptance and commitment therapy is the most recent addition to specific psychological treatments and is the nearest of these treatments to nidotherapy. But it has not been created as a treatment for personality problems but to help people manage common symptoms of mental illness such like anxiety and depression. Instead of cognitive restructuring or psychodynamic interventions to reorder and refocus attitudes, beliefs, and thoughts, acceptance and commitment therapy (ACT) concentrates on training people to accept unpleasant negative thoughts, feelings, symptoms, or situations without fighting them all the time. It also promotes more healthy ways of behaviour that are in keeping with the person's values, hopes, and goals.

The training in ACT helps develop a greater degree of psychological flexibility, the ability to discern long-term goals while still concentrating on the present. It is common in practice to think of the mantra 'Wake up, loosen up, and step up'. So instead of being preoccupied by troublesome feelings and symptoms, the patient is asked to reflect on what is important to them in life.

The 'loosen up' phase describes the 'willingness' of accepting any unpleasant feelings or symptoms. In a similar way to the treatment of phobias by immersion in the phobic situation; if the unpleasant feelings, be they anxiety, fear, depression, or emotional distress, are dispassionately accepted for what they are and given a more neutral status, they are better tolerated. The last phase, commitment, asks the patient to decide to concentrate on the goals already identified in phase one and how they are going to achieve these goals.

ACT (its inventors say it should be pronounced as one syllable) is described as a contextual behaviour therapy that allows for greater flexibility and is more geared to personal needs (Hayes, 2004; Hayes et al., 2006). We think it is admirably suited to the treatment of some personality disorders, particularly when mood disturbance is a primary feature, but to date there has been limited research examining its efficacy (Reyes-Ortega et al., 2020).

Other forms of treatment for personality disorder

STEPPS (Systems Training for Emotional Predictability and Problem-Solving)

STEPPS is a combined educational and therapeutic training programme focused on the emotional dysregulation of borderline personality disorder (Blum et al., 2002, 2008). It is a group treatment delivered over 20 sessions by two trained staff with experience in cognitive behaviour therapy and basic problem-solving. A randomised trial in outpatients showed greater improvements in impulsivity, negative affectivity, mood, and global functioning but no difference in suicidal behaviour or hospital admissions (Blum et al., 2008). Although these findings are not particularly impressive, the treatment has strong adherents.

A somewhat similar combined treatment, PEPS therapy (psycho-education combined with problem-solving), was found in a trial of nearly 200 patients with a range of personality disorders to be markedly superior to a waiting list control in terms of problem-solving skills, higher overall social functioning (the primary outcome), and anger expression (Huband et al., 2007). Because of the success of this initial study, a much larger one was planned with over 500 patients, a rigorous design, and generous funding from the National Institute of Health Research in the UK. If this had been completed successfully, it would have been the largest clinical trial of personality disorder treatment ever performed. Unfortunately, it had to be abandoned early because of adverse effects, including four people who died, two from suicide, in the active-treatment group. The treatment was highly structured, with a psycho-education module of up to 4 individual sessions and a problem-solving module of 12 sessions, each two hours long, to improve interpersonal problem skills. Three hundred and six patients were randomised, and it is unlikely the results would have been different if the trial had completed its full quota of participants. One of the concerns was that after completion of the interventions, therapy was not gradually tailed off, and this may have impacted the final results. One of the few positive results was a saving on total costs (McMurran et al., 2017), but in all **cost-effectiveness** studies, it is difficult to achieve significant differences because of large variations across patients.

One of the most lucid and thoughtful writers on the subject of personality disorders is Professor Joel Paris from McGill University in Montreal, Canada. He has written extensively about borderline personality disorder (Paris, 1996, 2003, 2020, 2025) and is a strong supporter of the diagnosis. To check on how much his views have changed since his first summary of the condition (1996), I asked him what has changed in the subsequent 28 years. Here are his two sets of responses:

I do not want to be a dampener of enthusiasm for a subject on which we have been far too pessimistic about treatment, but it is difficult to be proud of the achievements made in the last 28 years. There is also another treatment that needs to be considered with all the other specialised treatments. It is called structured clinical management in the UK (Bateman & Fonagy, 2009) and good (or general) psychiatric management in the US (Gunderson & Links, 2014; Choi-Kain et al., 2016). These treatments are said to be evidence based, but they are not. There have been no comparisons

Table 4.1 Joel Paris's nine-point summary of borderline personality disorder in 1996 and 2024

1996	2024
In the short term, there is relatively little change in borderline patients.	Even in the short term, we can see symptomatic remissions in these patients.
Recovery begins to become apparent after an average of 10 years.	But full recovery begins to become apparent later, as the brain continues to mature.
After 15 years, the majority of cases no longer meet diagnostic criteria for the disorder.	After 15 years, the great majority of cases no longer meet diagnostic criteria for this disorder.
Improvement is apparent in all aspects of the disorder but is most striking for impulsivity.	Improvement is apparent in all domains but is most striking for impulsivity.
Many patients, even when they no longer meet criteria for BPD, continue to have serious problems later in life and remain at risk of relapse.	Some patients, even when they no longer meet criteria for diagnosis, continue to have serious problems later in life.
A minority establish successful intimate relationships, but in most cases, improvement is associated with a withdrawal from intimacy.	Only about half achieve stable relationships, some withdraw from intimacy, and a significant minority are not stably employed.
About 10% of borderline patients eventually commit suicide.	Close to 10% of these patients eventually commit suicide, usually after failure to recover, but 90% do not (in spite of many attempts).
There are no clear-cut predictors of the outcome of BPD at baseline either for level of functioning or for suicide.	There are no clear-cut predictors of outcome at baseline, either for level of functioning or for suicide.
There is no evidence that treatment has an effect on long-term outcome.	While there are several evidence-based therapies for this population (especially DBT), we do not know the extent to which treatment has an effect on long-term outcome.

between these treatments and ordinary care that show them to be superior. Both structured clinical management and good psychiatric management involve working compassionately with the patient, their carers, and their families to build problem-solving skills and enable people to safely manage their emotions and behaviour. The aim is to enable them to live as independently as possible in their local community. It is not a short treatment; structured clinical management for individuals and their carers can last for up to two years. It is said to involve four phases—assessment, socialisation, treatment, and transition to ending. There are now courses taught in structured clinical management (SCM) to follow accepted fashion on the subject. It is now described at the Anna Freud Centre in London as

> an evidence-based approach that enables generalist mental health practitioners to work effectively with people with borderline personality disorder. SCM provides generalist mental staff with a coherent systematic approach to working with people with borderline personality disorder. It is based on a supportive approach with case management and advocacy support. There is an emphasis on problem-solving, effective crisis planning, medication review and assertive follow-up if appointments are missed. The new SCM Basic Training consists of 18 hours of instructor-led content over 3 days, and 21 hours of self-guided content.

All this sounds impressive, but where is its evidence base? It suggests that there is nothing of special significance in the input provided, but the fact that it runs very close to MBT in efficacy—the latest trial with suicidal attempts as the primary outcome showed more serious suicide attempts with MBT than SCM (Carlyle et al., 2020)—suggests that if all were successfully trained in basic good psychiatric management, we would have results to celebrate.

How do these treatments differ from basic community team practice? I cannot see any differences between sympathetic understanding, support during crises, sticking with therapy through difficult times, and ensuring regular follow-up, which should be the bedrock of good psychiatric care. It is certainly how I have attempted to practise throughout my professional life.

I want to make clear in writing this dismissal of borderline as a personality disorder that I am not in any way criticising the people who have been given this diagnostic label; I am just pointing out that the notion of borderline as a diagnostic entity is pseudoscience, so people who are so diagnosed are being cheated. One of the consequences of this pseudo-diagnosis is that treatment is being compromised. More than three-quarters of all people diagnosed with personality disorder are given the borderline diagnosis, but this includes a very large group that is heterogeneous. It includes people who have very severe emotional instability and pressing needs for treatment; many others have disorders that are best diagnosed differently and treated accordingly; another group has a mild degree of emotional dysregulation but many other problems that could be treated successfully; and a final group has no significant personality problems at all and is being diagnosed as borderline through spite, ignorance, or stigma.

It also needs to be made clear that the benefits of the intensive treatments described here are not particularly impressive. When Marsha

Linehan completed the development of dialectical behaviour therapy, she foresaw its progression in four stages. The first of these was the reduction of suicidal behaviour; the second was the building of better regulation of emotions so that distress, mood instability, and loneliness were reduced; the third was the creation of a more stable self; and the fourth, which she often called transcendence, was fulfilment of all needs in relationships. Without wanting to sound too gloomy, only the first of these and possibly part of the second have been shown to be effective.

Evidence-based medicine in this area sometimes comes in for a bit of a drubbing because anti-diagnosis is so prevalent. But it is the best lever we have to improve management of mental disorders. Even strong proponents of psychological treatment, such as Anthony Bateman and John Gunderson, together with Roger Mulder, were not too impressed by the findings. In their own review of treatment, they concluded,

> The evidence base for the effective treatment of personality disorders is insufficient. Most of the existing evidence on personality disorder is for the treatment of borderline personality disorder, but even this is limited by the small sample sizes and short follow-up in clinical trials, the wide range of core outcome measures used by studies, and poor control of coexisting psychopathology.
>
> (Bateman et al., 2015)

So we can safely conclude that we are only at first base when it comes to treatment.

If the highly specialised intensive treatments that we suspect from clinical trials are effective are applied to all the people who show variations on the borderline theme, there is bound to be confusion. The intended patients with severe emotional instability will be appropriately selected, but many of the others will receive these inappropriately or should never receive them at all. A bad diagnosis impairs research; the one that selects a homogeneous population is most appropriate for testing hypotheses. I suspect that many of the trials that have not shown particular benefits of specialised psychological treatments in borderline and other personality-disordered patients (e.g., Chanen et al., 2008; McMurran et al., 2017) could have yielded different results if the patients included had been selected with a different diagnostic system. I also think that the sad summary of a recent independent systematic review of the psychological treatment of borderline personality disorder tells us where we have gone wrong:

> The strength of evidence for the general effectiveness and comparative effectiveness of commonly used psychotherapies for the treatment of borderline personality disorder is mostly low to very low. The findings from

this systematic review suggest that all commonly used psychotherapies and treatment as usual improve borderline personality disorder severity, symptoms, and functioning, and there is no strong evidence suggesting that any one commonly used psychotherapy is more beneficial than another. In addition, very little is known about psychotherapy-related harms.

(Crotty et al., 2024)

This review contrasts with the more accepted opinion that all specialised treatments are effective (Choi-Kain et al., 2016) from the more biased viewpoints of their supporters. The reader is invited to come to a conclusion independently after comparing the data presented in these papers.

The winds of change are blowing, and it is likely that, by the time that this book is published, borderline and all the other categorical diagnoses that are still popular in the DSM system of classification will be abandoned in the same way that ICD-11 abandoned the categories of ICD–10. This could be followed by a better diagnostic description of emotional dysregulation that makes it clear where it differs from other conditions.

THE TREATMENT OF EMOTIONAL INSTABILITY

All the treatments described in the previous section are aimed at treating a personality disorder. I judge this to be wrong; in managing people with personality problems, we have to help them adapt but do this in the knowledge that we are not going to fundamentally change their personalities. The specific treatments for borderline personality disorder are trying to manage, adjust, or remove one aspect of the condition, emotional instability or dysregulation, which is not a personality domain. It is perfectly reasonable to focus on this very central element of the condition, but in doing so, it must be realised that the underlying personality is going to remain unaltered after completion of treatment. It does not mean that it will remain entirely unchanged. Many years ago, I suggested that personality disorders could be separated into immature and mature groups (Tyrer, 1988), with the immature one tending to improve over time. Those who are now diagnosed with borderline personality disorder are often in the immature personality group that will improve over time spontaneously, and this explains why some, but certainly not all patients improve dramatically when followed up for many years (Stone, 1993; Paris, 2003).

If many of the people who now are tagged with the label of borderline personality disorder were reassessed and the core group rediagnosed with emotional dysregulation disorder, we would then have a condition independent of personality that is ripe for treatment. It is not a personality domain; it is a highly unpleasant form of affective disorder (Tyrer, 2009) and needs focused treatment. The following suggestions are made to add focus to the treatment of those with prominent emotional instability that go beyond the specialist treatments already described. Please note that they are suggestions only and are made with little evidence.

Spend time alone   People with emotional instability have their most serious reactions after contact with other people. This is an obvious statement, but it will be clear that avoidance of other people might have some value. If you happen to be the only person on a desert island, you do not have many opportunities to demonstrate your emotional instability. If you can tolerate your own company, and I appreciate that sometimes this may be difficult, then a period away from other people, preferably spending time in an activity that you enjoy, can be very valuable. Sometimes, as Joel Paris (1996) has suggested, these people may be better without close relationships.

This is often called 'taking time out', but it is really taking time in, taking time to reassess your relationships with other people and determining who is likely to be able to help you and who is more likely to provoke you. Assessing this on your own can be an asset, as then you are not so likely to jump to solutions suggested by others who have a much shallower impression of your problems.

Manage the problem of identity   Identity disturbance is a key part of emotional dysregulation, but it is not well understood or adequately researched. It is 'characterized in large part by subjective distress (e.g. painful incoherence, self-hatred, feeling broken or evil) and private experiences (e.g. perceived discontinuities in, or incongruities between core beliefs/attitudes/values, feelings of derailment, feeling one lacks an identity)' (Kaufman & Meddaoui, 2021, p. 85), and these are not concepts that are easy to measure and assess over time. It is also not known if there are key qualitative elements of identity disturbance or whether it is best viewed as a spectrum.

One way, probably an unconscious one, that the nervous system manages identity disturbance is to switch over entirely to a new identity. This is a separate diagnosis, dissociative identity disorder. In this condition, there are two or more distinct personality states (dissociative identities), which are usually very different. (The classic fictional example is Robert Louis Stevenson's *Dr Jekyll and Mr Hyde*.) Each personality state includes its own pattern of relating to itself, its body, and the environment. Although complete dissociation of identity is not very common, it is of considerable interest as so many of the people who have the condition are reasonably well adjusted in their new personae and do not present for treatment. For many years, there was a supportive charity, First Person Plural, for people with this condition, usually abbreviated to DID. There is a partial form of the disorder, partial DID, in which there are only temporary breaks with the former personality, with one normally being dominant and being involved in most of the functions of daily life but which is every so often temporarily invaded by one or more of the non-dominant personality states (dissociative intrusions). At times these intrusive identities take over the personality and can affect behaviour (e.g., at times of extreme emotion, episodes of self-harm, or the recall of traumatic memories). In dissociative identity disorder, there is usually a complete separation of the personalities with amnesia for the alternative one (the alter ego), but this is not found in partial DID.

We do not yet know nearly enough about these dissociative states—they are elaborated on in cognitive analytical therapy—but better awareness of them might be helpful in managing emotional dysregulation, as the dissociation in these partial states does seem to have protective value and can reduce distress markedly.

Write it all down   The written word has its shortcomings, but it is a valuable record at times of distress. Memories of what you have done and said may be distorted in retrospect, unnecessarily magnified and exaggerated, but writing about all your experiences very soon after they have occurred can have a soothing and calming effect. The sentences you have written can be assessed when your mental state is more settled, and you are able to think logically. It is perhaps no coincidence that Marsha Linehan, in developing dialectical behaviour therapy, used the written word to regulate her thinking. In writing ' you can't think yourself into new ways of acting; you can only act yourself into new ways of thinking', she was emphasising that thought about actions was not enough on its own; she had to convert her own meaningful life experiences into a form that made sense, and writing about it led to the formulation of an effective treatment that could be replicated.

Similarly, Steven Hayes, in analysing his own experiences of recurrent panic attacks that led him to create acceptance and commitment therapy, realised that regarding negative emotions as ones that needed to be fixed, managed, or changed was not the right way forward; they had to be understood in the context of life. He wrote down his new thinking and its implications and rejected the notion that we should split our lives into parts that were favourable and parts that were toxic, then remove the toxic ones, and all would be hunky dory. Look on our own lives as problems to be solved, as if we can sort through our experiences for the ones we like and throw out the rest. He then developed the goal of ACT as greater acceptance of the context in which both positive and negative events happen.

The promotion of acceptance is also a key part of Marsha Linehan's DBT. This is a useful exercise: divide a sheet of paper with a line down the middle, entitle the left-hand part of the page as 'emotional events' and the right hand side as 'acceptance strategies'. So if the comment on the left is 'had bust up with Laura, felt suicidal afterward', the right-hand one could be 'we were both in a bad mood; we should have just recognised this and moved on'. Getting this down in writing helps, and you can come back to it again and again.

Keeping a diary may also help. It helps relieve emotional pressures and put them in a form where they can be neutralised. Anne Frank described this well in her diary: 'I can shake off everything as I write; my sorrows disappear, my courage is reborn'.

Take up acting   As already noted, people with emotional dysregulation can dissociate to escape from intolerable pressures. Just as an electrical circuit will cut out when placed in overload, our nervous systems do the same when the emotional input goes beyond the level we can tolerate. Dissociation is common when people are exposed to severe trauma. In extreme cases, the person not only separates his or her person from the traumatic situation but may also develop a completely different persona.

I am not suggesting that those who have such emotional disturbance should use dissociation as a form of management, even if it was possible, but a minor form of dissociation is achieved in drama. If you feel inadequate, useless, and unloved, with no-one recognising or respecting you, it is a boon to be transported into a role where you are a central figure, admired and copied for your abilities, and have a place of importance, even if this is only in play.

Set yourself an attainable goal   Goals are important in life; they are markers of progress. Those with emotional instability find many of their aims evaporate in the ether; they either fail or turn out to be illusory. But if you can set yourself clear, definable goals, whether in occupation, accommodation, or leisure achievements, and stick to them, they can remain as bright lights in the distance when you are struggling in the present.

Join a group of sufferers   One of the consequences of setting up services for borderline personality disorder is the failure to anticipate the flood of referrals. Most people who want treatment will never receive one of the highly specialised treatments discussed in this chapter and are very upset when their attempts to get treatment are deflected repeatedly to alternatives that are not wanted. Many who have emotional dysregulation are engaging and interesting people who readily meet with others who have similar problems. One of the advantages of forming a group who have similar problems is that all elements of stigma disappear, and you can talk honestly among yourselves about your symptoms and your reactions.

Polkinghorne (2004) has some harsh words about technology-driven scripts and program outlines as they prevent decisions that should be based on judgment. He argues that in psychological therapies, the process should not be driven by the requirements of an external treatment programme but by the dynamic interactions in therapy; 'effective decisions about what to do require a type of reasoning that is responsive to the specific aspects of a situation and sensitive to changes taking place in that situation' (Polkinghorne, 2004, p. 151).

If the technologically driven treatments for borderline personality disorder described here are not as important as we have previously thought, then this increases the scope of people with lived experience in developing interventions personal to them. Some of these are described in further detail in a book that is critical of current practice (Ramsden et al., 2020).

References

Akiskal HS, Chen SE, Davis GC, Puzantian VR, Kashgarian M, & Bolinger JM (1985). Borderline: an adjective in search of a noun. *Journal of Clinical Psychiatry*, 46, 41–48.

Antonovsky A (1979). *Health, Stress and Coping*. San Francisco: Jossey-Bass.

Bach B, Kramer U, Doering S, di Giacomo E, Hutsebaut J, Kaera A, et al. (2022). The ICD-11 classification of personality disorders: a European perspective on challenges and opportunities. *Borderline Personal Disorder and Emotional Dysregulation*, 9, 12.

Bateman A, Constantinou MP, Fonagy P, & Holzer S (2021). Eight-year prospective follow-up of mentalization-based treatment versus structured clinical management for people with borderline personality disorder. *Personality Disorders*, 12, 291–299.

Bateman A & Fonagy P (2009). Randomized controlled trial of outpatient mentalization-based treatment versus structured clinical management for borderline personality disorder. *American Journal of Psychiatry*, 166, 1355–1364.

Bateman A & Fonagy P (2016). *Mentalization-Based Treatment for Personality Disorders: A Practical Guide*. New York: Oxford University Press.

Bateman AW, Gunderson J, & Mulder R (2015). Treatment of personality disorder. *Lancet*, 385, 735–743.

Beck AT, Davis DD, & Freeman A (2015). *Cognitive Therapy of Personality Disorders* (3rd edition). New York: Guilford Press.

Beck AT, Freeman A & Associates (1990). *Cognitive Therapy of Personality Disorders*. New York: Guilford Press.

Blum N, Pfohl B, St. John D, Monahan P, & Black DW (2002). STEPPS: a cognitive-behavioral systems-based group treatment for outpatient clients with borderline personality disorder—a preliminary report. *Comprehensive Psychiatry*, 43, 301–310.

Blum N, St. John D, Pfohl B, Stuart S, McCormick B, Allen J, et al. (2008). Systems Training for Emotional Predictability and Problem Solving (STEPPS) for outpatient clients with borderline personality disorder: a randomized controlled trial and 1-year follow-up. *American Journal of Psychiatry*, 165, 468–478.

Carlyle D, Green R, Inder M, Porter R, Crowe M, Mulder R, et al. (2020). Randomized-controlled trial of mentalization-based treatment compared with structured case management for borderline personality disorder in a mainstream Public Health Service. *Frontiers in Psychiatry*, 11, 561916.

Chanen AM, Jackson HJ, Mccutcheon LK, Jovev M, Dudgeon P, Yuen HP, et al. (2008). Early intervention for adolescents with borderline personality disorder using cognitive analytic therapy: randomised controlled trial. *British Journal of Psychiatry*, 193, 477–484.

Choi-Kain LW, Albert EB, & Gunderson JG (2016). Evidence-based treatments for borderline personality disorder: implementation, integration, and stepped care. *Harvard Review of Psychiatry*, 24, 342–356.

Clarkin JF, Levy KN, Lenzenweger MF, & Kernberg OF (2007). Evaluating three treatments for borderline personality disorder: a multiwave study. *American Journal of Psychiatry*, 164, 922–928.

Crotty K, Viswanathan M, Kennedy S, Edlund MJ, Ali R, Siddiqui M, et al. (2024). Psychotherapies for the treatment of borderline personality disorder: a systematic review. *Journal of Consulting and Clinical Psychology*, 92, 275–295.

Davidson K, Norrie J, Tyrer P, Gumley A, Tata P, Murray H, et al. (2006). The effectiveness of cognitive behavior therapy for borderline personality disorder: results from the borderline personality disorder study of cognitive therapy (BOSCOT) trial. *Journal of Personality Disorders*, 20, 450–465.

Davidson KM, Tyrer P, Norrie J, Palmer SJ, & Tyrer H (2010). Cognitive therapy v. usual treatment for borderline personality disorder: prospective 6-year follow-up. *British Journal of Psychiatry*, 197, 456–462.

Giesen-Bloo J, Van Dyck R, Spinhoven P, Van Tilburg W, Dirksen C, Van Asselt T, et al. (2006). Outpatient psychotherapy for borderline personality disorder: randomized trial of schema-focused therapy vs transference-focused psychotherapy. *Archives of General Psychiatry*, 63, 649–658.

Gunderson JG & Links P (2014). *Handbook of Good Psychiatric Management for Borderline Personality Disorder*. American Psychiatric Publishing, Inc.

Gunderson JG & Singer MT (1975). Defining borderline patients: an overview. *American Journal of Psychiatry*, 132, 1–10.

Hayes SC (2004). Acceptance and commitment therapy and the new behavior therapies: mindfulness, acceptance, and relationship. In: SC Hayes, VM Follette, & MM Linehan (eds.), *Mindfulness and Acceptance: Expanding the Cognitive-Behavioral Tradition*. New York: Guilford Press.

Hayes SC, Luoma JB, Bond FW, Masuda A, & Lillis J (2006). Acceptance and commitment therapy: model, processes and outcomes. *Behaviour Research and Therapy*, 44, 1–25.

Huband N, McMurran M, Evans C, & Duggan C (2007). Social problem-solving plus psychoeducation for adults with personality disorder: pragmatic randomised controlled trial. *British Journal of Psychiatry*, 190, 307–313.

Jenkins G, Hale R, Papassatasiou M, Crawford M, & Tyrer P (2002). Suicide rate 22 years after parasuicide: cohort study. *British Medical Journal*, 325, 1155.

Kaufman EA & Meddaoui B (2021). Identity pathology and borderline personality disorder: an empirical overview. *Current Opinion in Psychology*, 37, 82–88.

Kernberg OF (2016). What is personality? *Journal of Personality Disorders*, 30, 145–156.

Krueger RF & Hobbs KA (2020). An overview of the DSM-5 alternative model of personality disorders. *Psychopathology*, 53, 126–132.

Lester R, Prescott L, McCormack M, & Sampson M; North West Boroughs Healthcare, NHS Foundation Trust (2020). Service users' experiences of receiving a diagnosis of borderline personality disorder: a systematic review. *Personality and Mental Health*, 14, 263–283.

Linehan MM (2015). *DBT Skills Training Manual*. Guilford Press.

Linehan MM, Armstrong HE, Suarez A, Allmon D, & Heard HL (1991). Cognitive-behavioral treatment of chronically parasuicidal borderline patients. *Archives of General Psychiatry*, 48, 1060–1064.

McMurran M, Day F, Reilly J, Delport J, McCrone P, Whitham D, et al. (2017). Psychoeducation and problem solving (PEPS) therapy for adults with personality disorder: a pragmatic randomized-controlled trial. *Journal of Personality Disorders*, 31, 810–826.

Mulder R & Tyrer P (2023). Borderline personality disorder: a spurious condition unsupported by science that should be abandoned. *Journal of the Royal Society of Medicine*, 116, 148–150.

Mulder RT, Horwood J, Tyrer P, Carter J, & Joyce PR (2016). Validating the proposed ICD-11 domains. *Personality and Mental Health*, 10, 84–95.

Mulder RT, Horwood LJ, & Tyrer P (2020). The borderline pattern descriptor in the International Classification of Diseases, 11th revision: a redundant addition to classification. *Australian and New Zealand Journal of Psychiatry*, 54, 1095–1100.

National Institute for Health and Care Excellence (2009). *Borderline Personality Disorder: Recognition and Management* (NICE Clinical Guideline CG78). London: NICE.

Paris J (1996). *Social Factors in the Personality Disorders: A Biopsychosocial Approach to Etiology and Treatment*. Cambridge University Press.

Paris J (2003). *Personality Disorders Over Time: Precursors, Course and Outcome*. American Psychiatric Publishing.

Paris J (2020). *Treatment of Borderline Personality Disorder, Second Edition: A Guide to Evidence-Based Practice*. Guilford Press.

Paris J (2025). *A Concise Guide to Borderline Personality Disorder*. American Psychological Association.

Paris J & Zweig-Frank A (2001). A 27-year follow-up of borderline patients. *Comprehensive Psychiatry*, 42, 482–487.

Polkinghorne DE (2004). *Practice and the Human Sciences: The Case for a Judgment-Based Practice of Care*. State University of New York Press.

Potter S (2020). *Therapy with a Map: A Cognitive Analytic Approach to Helping Relationships*. Pavilion.

Ramsden J, Prince S, & Blazdell J (eds.) (2020). *Working Effectively with 'Personality Disorder': Contemporary and Critical Approaches to Clinical and Organizational Practice*. Luminate (Pavilion Publishing and Media Ltd).

Reed GM (2018). Progress in developing a classification of personality disorders for ICD-11. *World Psychiatry*, 17, 227–229.

Reyes-Ortega MA, Miranda EM, Fresán A, Vargas AN, Barragán SC, Robles García R, et al. (2020). Clinical efficacy of a combined acceptance and commitment therapy, dialectical behavioural therapy, and functional analytic psychotherapy intervention in patients with borderline personality disorder. *Psychology and Psychotherapy*, 93, 474–489.

Ryle A (ed.) (1997). *Cognitive Analytic Therapy and Borderline Personality Disorder: The Model and the Method*. Chichester: Wiley.

Ryle A (2004). The contribution of cognitive analytic therapy to the treatment of borderline personality disorder. *Journal of Personality Disorders*, 18, 3–35.

Ryle A, Kellett S, Hepple J, & Calvert R (2014). Cognitive analytic therapy at 30. *Advances in Psychiatric Treatment*, 20, 258–268.

Sharan P, Das N, & Hans G (2023). Clinical Practice Guidelines for assessment and management of patients with borderline personality disorder. *Indian Journal of Psychiatry*, 65, 221–237.

Simmonds S, Coid J, Joseph P, Marriott S, & Tyrer P (2001). Community mental health team management in severe mental illness: a systematic review. *British Journal of Psychiatry*, 178, 497–502.

Stoffers-Winterling JM, Storebø OJ, Pereira Ribeiro J, Kongerslev MT, Völlm BA, Mattivi JT, et al. (2022). Pharmacological treatment for borderline personality disorder. *Cochrane Database of Systematic Reviews*, 1114, CD012956.

Stone MH (1993). Long-term outcome in personality disorders. *British Journal of Psychiatry*, 162, 299–313.

Tyrer P (ed.) (1988). *Personality Disorders: Diagnosis, Treatment and Course*. London: Wright.

Tyrer P (2009). Why borderline personality disorder is neither borderline nor a personality disorder. *Personality and Mental Health*, 3, 86–95.

Tyrer P (2013). From the Editor's desk. *British Journal of Psychiatry*, 202, 162.

Tyrer P (2024). *Intelligent Drug Prescribing in Psychiatry: Supporting the Patient-Prescriber Partnership*. CRC Press.

World Health Organisation (2024). *Clinical Descriptions and Diagnostic Requirements for ICD-11 Mental, Behavioural and Neurodevelopmental Disorders*. WHO: Geneva.

Young JE, Klosko JS, & Weishaar ME (2003). *Schema Therapy: A Practitioner's Guide*. Guilford Press.

Chapter 5

Understanding personality involves being honest with yourself

If you are to use nidotherapy to adapt your behaviour, your pattern of existence, and, in the longer run, your life to your personality, you need to be frank and open with yourself before starting the process. This does not mean you have to tell all others exactly what you are like, although a little disclosure seldom produces harm, but, when you have removed all the fluff and superficial coverings and got down to the bottom of who you really are, you can say with Shakespeare, 'to thine own self, be true'.

In the process of understanding, there are six aspects that should be considered, and the way they are accepted depends greatly on the dominant domains of your personality.

1. Be aware of your own personality at all times

This may seem obvious, but it isn't, and many people go through their lives blissfully ignorant of who they are or are perceived by others. Others create personalities they show to the world but know perfectly well they are phony; they are barriers to prevent others seeing what they are really like. A great deal depends on the domains that are dominant. Those with pronounced negative affective features are often acutely aware of their own personalities and exaggerate their deficiencies to an abnormal degree. The term I would like all to forget, borderline, takes in the full range of self-awareness—'one moment, I'm on top of the world, and the next, I'm drowning in self-doubt', and because these fluctuate so greatly, no satisfactory understanding is achieved. As a contrast, those with detached personalities often get on with their lives without ever considering who they are or where they are going. As understanding others is such a problem for them, it is not surprising they rarely analyse their own personal attributes. Charles Darwin was most comfortable working for long periods of time alone in his study, only getting up to go to the lavatory, which he did repeatedly, and often getting so preoccupied he forgot to drink or appear at meal times. He could engage with his frequent bodily complaints with

DOI: 10.4324/9781003560630-5

gusto but not with other people except at an analytical level. This did not mean he did not care about others, but because he was so bound up with his thoughts and theories, he thought of the people around him as peripheral figures in a more important intellectual existence.

Those in whom the anankastic domain dominates are also frequently full of self-doubt and over-analyse their feelings and attitudes. They are often accurate in assessing their personalities but spend long periods ruminating about them without ever reaching a solution. Being bound up with nothing is but what is not, like the musings of Macbeth, can become a circular nightmare.

People who are disinhibited often do understand their personalities, but this does not necessarily change their behaviour. We all know of people who, at times of particular stress or disruption in their lives, behave 'out of character' and act in a way that is completely contrary to their normal behaviour. This does not imply that such behaviour is necessarily maladaptive—the nervous junior who finally stands up to his bullying boss can often turn the tables in the relationship—but we need to be aware that these temporary events are anomalies and take us out of our personality comfort zones.

This does not mean we need to be constantly aware of who we are and so become embarrassingly self-absorbed. The important question we need to ask ourselves in these circumstances is simple: 'Is this really me, and why am I different from the way I normally am?' If you go outside the areas where your normal personality usually resides, you need to know why. 'Do I need to review my comfort zone?' is the current expression (even though to me it is a familiar armchair). Being unaware and ploughing on in unfamiliar territory will make you uncomfortable and lead to problems.

2. Do not believe that your personality will change fundamentally

One of the reasons the term 'personality disorder' has had such a bad press is that it is regarded as a permanent feature of the person concerned. The implication is that you do not have an external disorder afflicting you; the disorder is you—you, nasty person, are the disorder, and so you cannot escape.

The germ of truth in this damning conclusion is that the average person with very few personality problems has what Antonovsky (1979) calls a 'sense of coherence', in which the persona is completely in tune with his or her internal and external environments, recognises the reasons to engage with them, and has the resources to do so. As a consequence, people with a strong sense of coherence sail through life with very few perturbations, and their personalities do not alter very much over time.

Those with some degree of personality difficulty—and by now most readers will realise they cannot pretend they are free from this—can only achieve this sense of coherence by hard work in adjusting both internal and external environments to bring the sense of coherence back to an optimum level.

But the really important message to get over is that with this adjustment, which throughout this book is reworded as adaptation, those who might formerly have been classified as disordered can return to normal function and lose the status of both disorder and difficulty. So this explains why personality disorder is so unstable over time, especially when it is identified in younger people. In our own 30-year follow-up study of people with anxiety and depression, more than half changed their personality status (as measured by a standard instrument) over the follow-up period, and almost all who did not change had no personality problems at baseline (Yang et al., 2022). It is only the people who have no need to change their personalities who stay the same over time. Successful adaptation does not involve a change in your personality structure; it just makes a better fit to setting and so corrects the imbalance that previously was damaging.

3.   Chronicle all those occasions when you have felt fully in tune with your environment

Le us assume that everybody who feels they have a personality problem had a period in the past when this problem either did not exist or was present at a very low level. This can be an important clue to resolution. I am currently trying to help somebody who is persistently stuck in the negative affective domain of her personality and has been for nearly 80 years. She sees the whole of life through a lens of anxiety and threat and has done since the age of four. But she had a period when she was married before her husband died when she lost her worries almost entirely. We are trying to recreate these same past circumstances in one form or another as part of her management.

Of course we also have to acknowledge that some people may feel they have never felt comfortable with their personalities at any time in their lives, and so this exercise may be of no value.

Consider all the possibilities of making change with the least disruption to your personal wishes.

4.   Identify each personality difficulty and the environments in which it most manifests

This is not a difficult task, and it is particularly useful for those who feel they have personality difficulty and nothing more. Because those who have such difficulties are perfectly well adjusted most of the time, it is easy to forget, or remember only to dismiss, the times when you are at your worst. When I was at (a boys') school, I, like most others, joined the Combined Cadet Force, a preparation for national service as, at the time, it was expected all would be called up after leaving school. One of the tasks I was asked to do in front of all the other boys in the Force was to assemble a Bren gun. Most readers will not have seen a Bren gun, but it is a bit of military equipment that frightens you just to look at it—every part is menacing. It certainly frightened me, and attempting to fit it into its lethal operational form was quite beyond me, even after the briefest of demonstrations beforehand. But I persisted, over and over, pathetically trying to join up bits of metal with extraordinary shapes while hearing quiet sniggers in the background. Eventually I threw it down and said, 'This is ridiculous'. There was shock followed by laughter, and I heard someone say to another boy, 'Its difficult to believe, isn't it? I hear he's quite good at his lessons'.

This experience can easily be recorded as one of the slings and arrows of outrageous fortune that all of us come across at some time or another, but this exposed my personality difficulties. I subsequently spent hours practising the assembly of Bren guns until I could do this in my sleep and yet went through a long period when I could not face my fellow pupils as I was so humiliated. A person without my personality problems would have shaken this off with a laugh and a joke; I suffered for it.

Most of us will have had experiences like this, in which we have felt exposed at a weak point. I have met many people who have not progressed at work because they are terrified of formal job interviews, feeling they will be turned down for trivial omissions and errors. So they trundle on in their old roles, feeling undervalued and complaining that they are not appreciated, when just a bit of courage and grit could change their positions very easily. Those with obsessional personality features are particularly liable to these fears, expecting the worst and rehearsing it over and over in their minds.

5. Look for the environments that best compensate for or nullify the personality difficulty

There are always times in which unsettled people can feel the sense of coherence that all is going well. These may be brief and unable to persist, but sometimes, they can be expanded into a different lifestyle. In the past, I was involved in assessing the people with the most severe personality disorders in England, people with so-called 'dangerous and severe personality disorder'. No such condition actually exists; it was one decided by government diktat, but it did lead to a more humane approach to treatment in many prisons (see Chapter 11). One of the people we saw (he had committed a particularly brutal murder) had ready access to the library in the prison where he had been placed. He was not a person who had read much in the past, and the ready access to the well-stocked library in the prison was an eye-opener for him.

He spent more and more of his spare time in the library and then decided to start writing himself. When we assessed him, he had no desire to leave the prison. He was involved with a complex set of psychological interventions that very few could understand, and he asked to have these extended as much as possible so he could stay close to his beloved library. At an unexpected time in his life, he had found contentment.

There are many others who will have experiences that chime with this. The memories of a certain holiday when everything went right, the meeting with a person who had all the promise of a soulmate, the part-time job which made you feel as one with the world all can be treasured and remembered. Examine why these experiences were so positive for you and see if you can build on them.

6.   Be honest with yourself and admit any personality difficulties, even if your never share them with others

This is the most difficult of these six aspects of understanding. Approximately eight out of ten people have some difficulties with their personalities. The Arthurs of this world are in a minority; the rest of us have to puzzle a little. Most of the time, we do not think of our problems in relationships as having much to do with our personalities. Those with emotional stability at the core of these problems are the exception; they blame themselves and others in equal measure and go through much soul-searching. One of the main components of successful treatment here is what Marsha Linehan calls 'radical acceptance', which she defines as 'complete and total acceptance, from deep within, of the facts of reality. It involves acknowledging facts that are true and letting go of a fight with reality' (Linehan, 2015, p. 417). A distinction has to be made between beliefs that are usually based on supposition and facts that are true. So the belief that 'Maria hates me because she completely ignored me when I spoke to her' has to be counteracted by the fact that 'Maria is deaf and did not hear what I said, so that is why she seemed to snub me'. It is sometimes much easier to let beliefs take over from facts because they seem to fit the emotions, but they are poor guides.

At the opposite extreme are people, almost certainly ones who would never read books like this, who blame all their difficulties with people on others. They completely fail to recognise that their own behaviour and actions are the main reasons for their problems with others and absolutely deny the obvious conflict they create. This can become particularly serious when the person concerned wields a great deal of power. Josef Stalin, dictator of Russia for 29 years, was a grossly suspicious man who was probably responsible for up to 60 million deaths since he assumed power. Any form of criticism, heard, seen, implied, or suspected, was enough for you to be executed or sent to the gulag. This extended to his personal life. Shortly before he died, he accused nine doctors of plotting to kill him. When he collapsed suddenly in his office, no doctor was called as all had been afraid of having anything to do with him, so there was nobody to attend to him as he lay unconscious on the floor, which he did for several hours. 'What loneliness is more lonely than distrust?' wrote George Eliot in her book *Middlemarch*. Josef Stalin, despite his affable Uncle Joe exterior, must have been a very lonely man.

Knowing your own personality will not necessarily keep you out of mischief, but it will make you think twice before making important decisions. When you read about successful people turning down invitations to take up important posts in politics, business, or the arts, it is not always a consequence of humility. It is often the recognition that parts of them that they would prefer others not to see might be exposed. So knowing your own personality could be a good protective device. Cultivate it if you can.

References

Antonovsky A (1979). *Health, Stress and Coping*. San Francisco: Jossey-Bass.
Linehan MM (2015). *DBT Skills Training Manual*. Guilford Press.
Yang M, Tyrer H, Johnson T, & Tyrer P (2022). Personality change in the Nottingham Study of Neurotic Disorder: 30 year cohort study. *Australian and New Zealand Journal of Psychiatry*, 56, 260–269.

Chapter 6

General principles of adaptation

Most people know about the famous theory of natural selection created primarily by Charles Darwin. This explains evolution by giving thousands of examples of animals and plants generating, thriving, and dying out at different time periods spread over thousands of years. The reason change takes place is a consequence of the environment changing, and if an organism does not adapt to the new environment, it will be snuffed out by others that are better adapted. Our planet would probably still be dominated by dinosaurs but for the catastrophic meteor strike 66 million years ago that wiped out most of the larger animals on Earth and gave space for the smaller ones to take over and evolve.

In Darwin's very first edition of his book *The Origin of Species*, this principle of adaptation was stated very clearly:

> The species that survives is the one that is able best to adapt and adjust to the changing environment in which it finds itself.

Unfortunately, this has been forgotten ever since the influential psychologist Herbert Spencer introduced the term 'survival of the fittest' after reading of Darwin's work. I challenged Richard Dawkins, the prolific Darwin defender, about this term when he gave a public lecture at Imperial College some years ago. I asked him, 'It is not more appropriate to use the term "survival of the adapted"? as these were the words in the first edition of his book'. His response was swift and brutal: 'He may have written it, but he didn't mean it'. But the principles of adaptation that are at the core of nidotherapy are much more appropriate than the notion of struggle for supremacy that is implied in 'survival of the fittest', a term that has been picked up by racial supremacists, big corporation bosses, and dictators over the years to justify their behaviour.

Darwin would have contradicted Dawkins. He contradicted Spencer when he wrote again later, '[I]t is not the strongest of the species that

DOI: 10.4324/9781003560630-6

survives, it is the one that is most adaptable to change'. Evolutionary change is a consequence of minor adaptations, mainly created by genetic variation, improving the reproductive success of an organism over thousands of generations and thereby creating a more dominant species. It is not the fittest that survive; it is the best adapted.

How do we apply the principles of adaptation to the much shorter span of a human life and the more rapid adjustments that are needed for success? The principles are the same, but where evolutionary advance depends on chance (Dawkins appropriately calls it *The Blind Watchmaker*) (Dawkins, 2015), the adaptation needed to achieve success in a single generation is best created by the person concerned. Most people with personality problems are in settings that are totally maladaptive; getting into adaptive ones needs a combination of thought and nidotherapy. But the adaptation has to be right for the individual, and the way in which it is undertaken has to take notice of their personality characteristics.

What are the ways in which we adapt to actions, behaviours, opinions, and situations that annoy us? I suggest we do this in six ways, all of which are highly relevant to nidotherapy.

1 **Confrontation**
   We identify the problem and tackle it head on.
2 **Avoidance**
   We get out of the way and avoid exposure to conflict whenever it appears.
3 **Leverage**
   We use the power we have to get what we want.
4 **Modification**
   We do everything possible to reduce the severity or the intensity of the adverse event, but, unlike leverage, there is nothing we ask for in return.
5 **Escape**
   We leave the situation and go elsewhere.
6 **Dissociation**
   We pretend the issue is of no matter and distract our minds into comfortable territory.

If you want to remember these six strategies, just think of the acronym CALMED.

Before we examine each of these with humans it is first useful to look at each of them with reference to plants, a subject that preoccupied Darwin much more than his more notable worries about the place of man in the evolutionary animal tree. Darwin was much happier examining the evolution of plants than the evolution of animals; this rarely led to conflict.

Confrontation: black walnut (*Juglans nigra*)

Some plants are very possessive of their positions and do not want any competition. Many trees do this by sending messages from their roots. One of the most aggressive of these is the black walnut, a tree that can grow to heights of 30 metres and lives for 200 years. It guards its position by producing toxic substances (phytotoxins) called juglones that inhibit the growth of most other plants, so when they are close to a black walnut, they wither and die. So you will seldom see other plants in the close vicinity of a black walnut. It has a permanent but invisible sign—Keep Out: Trespassers Will Be Poisoned.

Avoidance: marram grass (*Ammophila arenaria*)

There are many species of plants that avoid getting into competition with others by going to places no other plants would contemplate. If you have ever been walking on sand dunes, particularly close to the sea, you will come across clumps of a wiry grass seeming to grow entirely in the sand. This is marram grass, a grass that survives as it has both highly curved leaves that crowd together and prevent loss of water (through transpiration) and deep roots that go down into the sand to suck up the small amounts of water hidden there. So it thrives in desert conditions. There is no competition anywhere to be seen, just more clumps of marram grass.

Leverage: elegant sunburst lichen (*Rusavskia elegans*)

The most inhospitable continent is Antarctica. Flowering plants have a miserable time there—I once spent nearly two hours finding one of the two species in Deception Island close to the Antarctic Peninsula; it was a very insignificant grass. But there is one group of plants that has a strong presence in the continent, the lichens. There are over 200 of them there, and the sunburst lichen is a brilliant yellow exposition of them, a bright yellow representation on an otherwise featureless rock. Lichens combine green plants with fungi in an intimate relationship. The fungi absorb water and provide an anchor for the green algae, and in return, the algae make food from photosynthesis and feed the fungi. So the green algae have leverage over the fungi and vice versa. Both benefit by their offers to the other. Ideally, they would like to be independent, but in the environments inhabited by lichens, this is not an option.

Modification: sundew (*Drosera rotundifolia*)

Plants that grow in very acid peaty soil have one great desire; they want nitrogen. This is not easily released from the soil in which they grow, so they have developed a modification of their leaves; they are now fly killers. The round leaves secrete sticky dewdrops that attract small flies that are caught in the leaves and cannot escape. They die, and the nitrogen in their body parts is absorbed into the plant, a simple transfer of elements. Leaves have many properties, not always attractive and benign.

Escape: rosebay willow herb (*Chamaenerion angustifolium*)

The rosebay willow herb was often grown in gardens and orchards where its leaves were harvested to make herbal tea. But it is constricted in these settings and loves to escape into open spaces, especially to ground that has recently been disturbed and is exposed. So it loves colonizing areas where the ground cover has been burnt. (In America, it is called fireweed.) It is a great favourite of rail passengers, first looking at newly created grey embankments and six months later seeing them festooned in the pinkish glory of a country fairground. This is a plant that starts scruffy but always escapes into glory.

Dissociation: bluebell (*Hyacinthoides nonscripta*)

Some plants gloriously ignore any of the negative elements of the settings in which they grow and throw away their doubts and fears. The bluebell is one of them. Its favourite place is deciduous woodland, often amongst dense-packed trees that for most of the year are drab, dank, and disinteresting. But for a few weeks in late spring, the woodland becomes a forest of nodding blue flowers, a pure, unadulterated, and intense blue that has few competitors anywhere else in the artistic world. This is floral dissociation at its best.

Let's move back to humankind. Does your personality have an influence on which of these strategies you employ in dealing with adaptation? By golly, it does—it's the prime mover.

Put yourself in the following situation and see how you would respond. You are at a meeting where you are sitting at the back of a room. It is quiet at first, and then you hear a loud drilling in the room behind you. It is difficult to hear what is going on at the meeting. What do you do? Think of the CALMED acronym. You could adopt any one of these strategies; your personality usually determines the one you choose.

Confrontation: You either get the organisers of the meeting to ask the obstreperous driller to stop working while the meeting is on, or you leave the room and let the driller know yourself. Your expression and hidden threat will *make him obey*.

Avoidance: Although the noise is very loud in your ears, it does not bother the people sitting farther forward, so you get up and move to a seat much nearer to the front. The drilling sound continues, but you can hear all that is going on at the meeting.

Leverage: You or the organisers go and see the drill man and come to an arrangement for the times he should stop and start drilling again.

Modification: You are a considerate person and realise the poor man has a
  job to do. You slip out to the room behind and ask the driller to work
  on a different part of the wall that makes the sound less marked in the
  meeting room.

Escape: The meeting is not that important. You can't hear anything; its not
  worth the candle. So you get up and leave.

Dissociation: You can't be bothered to kick up a fuss. You retreat into an
  oasis of calm inside your head. You can't hear much of the meeting, but
  as you have switched off, the noise loses its intensity and impact.

In this set of options, we only have one event. But those who have personality problems have a whole series of them extending for years. This sequence
shows the different parts of adaptation in a nutshell. But it only covers a
short period; to adapt to your personality effectively may take half a lifetime.

At different times in a person's life, the strategies of adaptation may be
different and also may need a combination of approaches. But some personalities will eschew some the six options here permanently because they
are antithetic to their inner personality structures. For example, I know
many we have come across in nidotherapy who avoid any form of confrontation. It is just considered alien as their personalities are the antitheses of
conflict—they force themselves to fit in with others' views, no matter how
odd they seem to be.

In the course of my clinical practice, I have come across the phenomenon called folie à deux—the sharing of delusional beliefs—in which one
of the individuals is suffering from a delusion, and the other believes it also
despite not having any form of psychosis. In both my encounters, the party
with no illness was a sister who was heavily reliant on her dominant psychotic sibling, so it was very easy to see how she would naturally soak up
all the psychotic beliefs of her sister and promulgate them as her own. Similarly, there are others, whom we shall be examining in a later chapter, who
are far too organised—some might use the word *obsessional*—to use the
escape option. It is seen as full of uncertainty and therefore full of danger.

The importance of personality strengths and domain traits in adaptive strategies

Judging the need for adaptation

In evolutionary terms, the need for adaptation depends on whether the
environmental changes are long term. If they are short term only (e.g., a
drought or a flood), the species may lose some members, but others will
survive and multiply once conditions improve again. The same applies
in nidotherapy but over a much shorter time period. If there is an unexpected event in any aspect of the environment, such as illness, an accident,

Table 6.1 Strategies of adaption separated by trait domains

	Negative affectivity	Detachment	Disinhibition	Dissociality	Anankastia
Adaptive strategy	Dissociation	Avoidance	Escape	Confrontation	Modification & leverage
Main strength	Emotional awareness	Independence	?	Determination	Caution

a change in a relationship, or a financial disturbance, then there may be no need to make any changes; you hunker down and hope for the best.

If a person is quite certain about his or her life's course, there is no need for external advice or intervention. This is why nidotherapy principles apply to everybody. We choose whom we spend most of our time with, what work we do, and what leisure interests we have and plan our futures accordingly. We only need or seek (and these are not the same, as often those who need and never seek and vice-versa) when the balance of life goes askew, and we lose our bearings.

I finish this chapter with an example from our work over the past 20 years. This illustrates how nidotherapy uses the principles of adaptation to get a life back on an even keel or, in this particular example, create an even keel when there was only a rocky road before. This is a personal statement from a patient, Heather Cameron, from Prince Edward Island, Canada, who was introduced to nidotherapy by my colleague and friend Dr Ben Spears in 2012, after he attended one of our nidotherapy workshops. Her words, which also appear on our website—www.nidotherapy.co.uk—are reproduced exactly as she has written them and with her consent, and I add my own comments in italic text for explanation at different points. Her account also illustrates each of the six strategies for adaptation at different times.

My name is Heather, I am sixty two and have suffered with mental health issues most of my life. It wasn't until my doctor introduced nidotherapy in 2012 that I finally felt relief.

I was bullied by an older sibling as child which manifested in day terror dreams as I grew older. Looking back, I can see that I was depressed when I was in my last year of University.

I was in my late twenties when symptoms of depression reoccurred. My brother died in July 1987 and then in January 1988 I quit my job with the excuse that I was going to travel in Europe. I did go to Europe for 5 weeks but there was no need to quit my job. After my trip I couldn't look for work. I had all kinds of thoughts that I wasn't good enough, no one would want to hire me and I didn't even have the confidence to ask for an application form. I finally decided I should see my doctor. She asked me if I could push a button that would end my life would I push it? I said yes. She referred to a Community Mental Health Clinic where I saw a psychologist.

The psychologist referred me to a psychiatrist who worked in the clinic. The psychiatrist prescribed an antidepressant and I would take a handful at bedtime and hope I wouldn't wake up. I knew nothing about drugs or quantities so I would wake up in the morning feeling fine. My psychologist got wind of this so on April 9, 1990 at the age of 29 I was admitted to the psychiatric ward at the local hospital and that evening I met Dr. Spears for the first time. He has been with me through everything and saved my life by introducing me to nidotherapy via NIDUS-UK. *[The account up to this point shows that Heather had serious psychiatric problems that were not temporary.]*

Dr. Spears tried everything with me: ECT, all kinds of medication, referred me to different counsellors, hospitalisation on PEI [Prince Edward Island] and away from PEI, DBT and CBT groups, including his own group therapy group and hours of psychotherapy. I might have short periods of feeling well but nothing lasted. I had numerous suicide attempts and suicide ideation was always there. The thought of suicide gave me hope.

I cut up, put ligatures around my neck, tried to choke on gobstoppers, tried to hook a hose to the exhaust pipe of my car, took overdoses of pills and tried to hang myself once when I was in hospital. I was also a binge eater as I saw this as a way of punishing myself. *[Heather describes her low self-esteem and her serious suicide risk; many of the interventions were introduced to stave off suicidal intent.]*

I arrived at Dr. Spears office with my dog, on a Saturday morning in May 2012 after a suicide attempt the night before. He drove me to the hospital and then took my dog home. When he got to my home the family was gathered inside having a merry time. That was his epiphany moment. He saw incongruity between what was going on with me and the family. *[Dr Spears had not been to the family home before, and what he saw there opened his eyes to the environment there. Heather was seen as a pathetic milksop, someone who was never going to change and whose influence on the family was negligible.]*

After discharge from hospital he broached the subject with me of having my own place. My living at home with my parents had always been an unquestioned arrangement for emotional and other reasons.

I was very receptive to the idea, so Dr. Spears started with nidotherapy. The first step was to tell my parents. I didn't feel able to do that so Dr Spears facilitated that by meeting with my mother and my sister. *[Here we introduce confrontation and avoidance. Heather had never been able to challenge her parents about leaving home and had always avoided the subject to 'keep the peace'. But Dr Spears had to confront the need for Heather to move. By putting nidotherapy into the context of a medical intervention and reassuring the family that their fears of suicide if she was on her own were unwarranted, he was able to get their agreement for Heather to leave.]*

He was able to reassure my mother that she wasn't losing me and that he thought my health would benefit from this move. *[Here we have leverage being implemented. If Heather was allowed to leave, she would not break off contact and still have regular contact with the family. Both parties would benefit.]* The next step was to help me get an apartment. I couldn't afford an apartment on my disability pension. Dr Spears was able to call in a favour and enable me to get a subsidy for an apartment. *[Leaving the family home for independent living was a good idea in principle, but it had to be implemented in practice. Here we see modification in play, with Dr Spears using his contacts to get supportive accommodation and a grant.]*

The moment I found out I had received a grant I started to feel better. It was several months before I was able to find an apartment but I was already feeling well. *[Heather has truly escaped. She has repeatedly said that as soon as she left home with the prospect of independence, she would be better.]* I can remember walking down a street and realizing I was smiling. That would happen frequently. I lost weight, became more involved my church volunteering on several committees. I started working on my own doing home care. I would often receive referrals from Dr. Spears of people who would need mental health support. *[Dissociation may not be the best way of describing Heather's feelings, but everyone has noticed she is a completely different person with a confident and secure persona. She is truly dissociated from her past existence.]*

It has now been 10 years since I left home and I still feel great. I have dealt with the death of my father and a beloved dog. I have had strife in the family with a sister who has caused a lot of mental pain but I have never thought of cutting up or over dosing or giving up on life as I would have before my nidotherapy intervention. *[Heather continues to help in supporting other patients in the acute phase of illness and her complete recovery—complete is the accurate adjective here—has been a spur to others currently in despair.]*

Heather Cameron, Charlottetown,
Prince Edward Island, Canada
December 2022

It is also fair to add that Heather now has no traces of personality disorder anywhere in her psyche; a fuller account of her experiences has been published (Spears et al., 2017). At the time this paper was submitted for publication, one of the referees doubted that her account was accurate as nobody with 'such a past history of personality pathology could possibly have recovered completely'. I wish I could introduce Heather to this reviewer now; he would be convinced.

References

Darwin C (1859). *On the Origin of Species by Means of Natural Selection, or the Preservation of Favoured Races in the Struggle for Life.* John Murray.

Dawkins R (2015). *The Blind Watchmaker: Why the Evidence of Evolution Reveals a Universe Without Design.* W.W. Norton.

Spears B, Tyrer H, & Tyrer P (2017). Nidotherapy in the successful management of comorbid depressive and personality disorder. *Personality and Mental Health*, 11, 344–350.

Chapter 7

Why nidotherapy can help adaptation

To understand how nidotherapy can help adaptation to personality problems, it is necessary to understand the principles behind it. In this chapter, I may repeat myself at times, but I need to get the message home.

As already described, there are ten basic principles of nidotherapy, but I do not apologise for repeating them (Box 7.1).

Box 7.1. Ten principles of nidotherapy

1 All people have the capacity to improve their lives when placed in the right environment.
2 Everyone should have the chance to test themselves in environments of their own choosing.
3 When people become distressed without apparent reason, the cause can often be found in the immediate environment.
4 A person's environment includes not only place but also other people and self.
5 Seeing the world through another's eyes gives a better perspective than your eyes alone.
6 What someone else thinks is the best environment for a person isn't necessarily so.
7 All people, no matter how disabled or handicapped, have strengths that can be fostered.
8 A person's environment should never be regarded as impossible to change.
9 Every environmental change involves some risk, but this is not a reason to avoid it.
10 Mutual collaboration is required to change environments for the better.

DOI: 10.4324/9781003560630-7

The reason these principles are particularly important in the adaptation of personality disorders is that all of them are linked to autonomy, the freedom from external control, and so many who have personality disorders have lost this autonomy.

Principle 1. Improvement in the right environment

This may look like a mom and apple pie statement because it seems so obvious. But it is not obvious at all. Even the best of us make mistakes in choosing what we think is the right environment, and often we have to try several times to get the right one. Many of those with personality problems have lost confidence in their ability to choose how to better their lives, and simple suggestions will not do. It helps enormously if people can make a proper analysis of their personality from the advice in Chapter 5 as, if this is done successfully, a good environmental change can be made. But no one can claim this is easy. I do not think I understood my personality fully until middle age, and most of the people who want advice are much younger than that. So when people have decided what the right environment is for them, it should be carefully dissected for snags and problems before it is followed through. But once it is followed through, it is owned by the person concerned, not the nidotherapist.

Principle 2. Everyone should have the chance to test themselves in environments of their own choosing

Far too often, people are asked to make a leap in the dark when making changes in their lives. If there is the opportunity to test options, they should always be taken. One of the reasons our clinical trial of nidotherapy was successful in keeping patients out of hospital (Ranger et al., 2009) was that we always took the option of testing out placements after discharge for a short period before making a final decision.

Principle 3. When people become distressed without apparent reason, the cause can often be found in the immediate environment

We introduced this principle after using nidotherapy to treat people with intellectual difficulty who were not always able to articulate what was concerning them. But this principle is relevant in personality disorders also. The manifestation of unexpected aggression in an alien environment, such as an acute admission ward in crisis, is a classical example.

Principle 4. A person's environment includes not only place but also other people and self

This is repeated so often elsewhere in this book it does not need amplification here.

Principle 5. Seeing the world through another's eyes gives a better perspective than your eyes alone

This principle also might appear to be self-evident. But this has to be seen against the history of medical professionals making decision after decision about the future of patients seen entirely from their personal point of view. Whatever the patient feels or says in these situations is usually ignored. The assumption is made that mental illness has prevented rational thought, and their solutions to problems are distorted and disarrayed, so they can readily be ignored. At the very least, the person giving advice in nidotherapy has to explore why the views of the patient are the way they are and whether there is an internal logic in their wishes that needs to be developed to find appropriate solutions.

Principle 6. What someone else thinks is the best environment for a person isn't necessarily so

This is the opposite side of the coin from Principle 5 and can often involve the nidotherapist in many hours of environmental advocacy. It is very easy in a mental health system to overrule the wishes of patients because they interfere with the plans incorporated into that system. This creates a set of false logical processes—our system operates in an agreed and accepted way; the patient is presenting an alternative way that clashes with our system; because our system is an agreed consensual one involving all, then, by definition, the patient's views are contradictory and therefore can be overruled. The rule that good management always involves listening to the consumer is overlooked.

Principle 7. All people, no matter how disabled or handicapped, have strengths that can be fostered

One of the common assumptions that practitioners make in assessing and helping people with personality disorders is that all those affected are inherently vulnerable and have weaknesses. This is assumed wrongly, mainly because strengths are never addressed in the assessment. But personality strengths can overcome apparent weaknesses and help create a compensated personality in which the weaknesses are hidden and may never be exposed.

We have developed a simple assessment of personality strengths that we have found useful when helping people overcome problems associated with their personality (Yang et al., 2022). We are sure that many others could be developed—there is an excellent one for assessing strengths in children (Goodman, 1997)—and one is needed specifically for those with personality disorders.

Principle 8. A person's environment should never be regarded as impossible to change

There are a few circumstances in which environmental change is very difficult, if not impossible, particularly if your life is controlled by external agencies (e.g., incarceration), but when you consider all the different ways in which shifts can be made in the many aspects of social, personal, and physical settings, the word 'impossible' can be dropped. People with personality problems sometimes feel that all the outlets for change have been blocked off; it is the task of nidotherapy to show that this is not so.

Principle 9. Every environmental change involves some risk, but this is not a reason to avoid it

We are unfortunately living in a highly risk-averse society in which actions of great worth and good intent are often inhibited by an infinitesimal chance of risk. There are many case examples in this book in which the required changes would never been made if the clarion call of risk had been sounded. I was warned when I first came down to London as a consultant that home visits were too risky, and I should avoid them. The only time I was assaulted was at the hospital unit (by an angry young man because I would not allow his girlfriend to leave). The most productive of all my nidotherapy encounters were at home.

Principle 10. Mutual collaboration is required to change environments for the better

As well as following these principles, there is a standard process that is used in nidotherapy. But as nidotherapy is a collaborative process that varies between many individuals deciding on their environmental changes with very little input and a much smaller group that need a great deal of support and help to achieve their aims, it is not necessary for this advice to be followed slavishly. The essential element in this area is mutual trust; if both patient and therapist are seen to be doing their best in good faith, any obstacles along the way can be overcome.

Phase 1. Understanding the person

There are four essential phases in nidotherapy. The first involves getting a full understanding of the person needing help as well as their environmental wishes. If, of course, the person is organising most of the aspects of environmental change themselves, this phase of nidotherapy is already covered. But if an external person is acting as a nidotherapist, there has to be a period before any decisions are made in which both the nidotherapist and the patient are fully at ease with each other and in a position of mutual trust. It is well established that the ability to engage with people in a way that is honest, genuine, and empathic is a core feature of all good psychotherapy. But it is possible for these words to trip off the tongue too readily; trust involves the ability to openly disagree and to come to compromises. The nidotherapist is trying to find out exactly what it feels like to be the patient within the framework of their lives and what seems to be necessary to change. The term 'collateral collocation' was given to this phase when nidotherapy was first formulated in the first book on the subject (Tyrer, 2009). For many professionals, the process of approaching patients' problems in the very personal way they are seeing them is difficult. It is a process of levelling down that is also being practised by another new approach called open dialogue, based on family systems therapy, which approaches patients in the same way as nidotherapy by 'facilitating autonomy and transparent decision-making' (Tribe et al., 2019). In meetings with open dialogue, both clinicians and patients express their feelings with greater self-disclosure and expression of emotions than is found in ordinary practice, and sometimes this can make patients feel uncomfortable. The principle of nidotherapy, 'seeing the world through another person's eyes', is the principle that needs to be remembered whenever there appears to be a mismatch between how the patient and the therapist view the same problem. Some might say it is impossible to removal all elements of authority and status from a person who has been trained to have greater knowledge and ability, but it is not necessary to flaunt these as evidence of superiority.

Phase 2. Environmental analysis

Psychoanalysis is a highly complex subject that some people study all their lives without fully comprehending its range. This is not surprising as the functioning of the mind still remains a closely guarded secret proudly protected in the depths of the brain. Environmental analysis is much easier, and in nidotherapy, it can sometimes be very straightforward indeed (see Heather's account in Chapter 6). At other times, it can be incredibly complex because many needs of equal importance can be identified, but often, these overlap or contradict each other, and it is far from clear what the patient actually wants and needs. We often have to consider all elements of the environment. It covers the full range of physical options from the country in which you live to the furniture in your kitchen, a similar range of social options involving very large or very small numbers of people with very different personalities and motivations, and the final set of personal environmental requirements that could be summarised as feeling good in your own skin.

If the therapist is able to understand the personality of the person who is having environmental concerns, the solutions become easier to find. In the first paper published on nidotherapy (Tyrer, 2002), I described the case of a 33-year-old Afro Caribbean woman, Mavis, whose husband had left home and left her to look after her three children alone. She tried hard but was unable to cope with her responsibilities, and they were taken into care. She became more reclusive and uncommunicative and was felt to be developing schizophrenia. I saw Mavis for the first time at an assessment for compulsory admission—never the best time to have your first contact with a patient—and when she tried to attack the social worker with an iron bar, we all felt admission under section was correct. (The iron bar was not mentioned in the case report.) But after admission and, we thought at the time, the prescription of antipsychotic drugs, she became much more approachable and explained her distress and anger at the social worker because, in her mind, this profession only existed to take her children away, and, when it came to the last of the three, she felt she had to put up a fight.

Mavis was placed in a hostel with other residents and did not get on well with them or the staff. To most of them, she was known as the 'iron bar woman' and therefore possessed of powerful antisocial tendencies. This was quite mistaken, and the more I got to know her, the more gentle she appeared. What she found particularly annoying was the heavy monitoring of her activities, and as she responded to these by angrily saying they were unnecessary, she was monitored even more frequently. It became increasingly clear to me that she did not have a psychotic illness but was a person with a very detached personality structure who largely preferred her own company and did not desire or need the presence of others. After a great deal of negotiation—now called environmental advocacy in nidotherapy—she was placed for a trial period in a low-staffed hostel which had a standard policy of one visit each week from a support worker and a full review every six months; the rest of the time, the residents were allowed to live their own lives.

This proved to be remarkably successful. Not only did Mavis blossom in this low-supervised residence, but after a few months, she was able to persuade her social worker to let her have contact with her children again, and by the time I ceased my contact with her, she was seeing them almost every week. By then, we had been able to stop all her medication.

The key to understanding Mavis's environmental needs was her personality assessment. She responded very badly to monitoring of her behaviour, no matter how sensitively it was carried out, as it was perceived not as a friendly check-up but as an intrusion. Once this understanding was reinforced by extra evidence that she was competent at looking after her own affairs, it was a relatively stress-free passage from that time on. By having a better understanding of her personality and the reasons for some of her aggressive behaviour, it was also possible to review her diagnosis, reduce her medication for the original diagnosis of paranoid schizophrenia, and subsequently stop all her medication. I cannot be certain, but I think it would be highly unlikely that, if I had used standard practice without assessing Mavis's personality, this positive long-term outcome would have been achieved.

Phase 3. Setting the timetable for environmental change

Although some environmental changes can be made quickly and smoothly, those involving personality disorder usually have to be made more slowly. In setting a timetable for the implementation of the environmental change, much needs to be made of the need to accommodate the personality at the same time. For a number of reasons, many of those with personality problems get stuck in a circle of despond when nothing seems to go right. Some of these have what I describe as the Prufrock syndrome, illustrated in the next chapter, while others, particularly those with strong elements of the detached and anankastic domains, find all sorts of reasons why possible change cannot be effected. In our 30-year study of patients with anxiety and depressive disorders, those who had a personality disorder at the outset of the study were much less likely to experience a positive environmental change over the 30-year period of follow-up (Tyrer et al., 2021). They were also significantly less likely to make occupational changes over the 30-year period than those with no personality disorder. It was almost as though the expectation of change had been drummed out of them many years earlier, and they doggedly continued in the same environmental prison that had been created for them. It is in these situations that the principles of environmental advocacy have to be brought to the fore. Often, the patient wants to see a change but is pessimistic about it being achieved and, at times, almost self-sabotages any direction of change. I am still, with colleagues, trying to help a person who is quite capable of working, but every single attempt to get a successful work placement is given up at a very early stage. Part of this concern is generated by the anxiety of returning to work after many years, but some is generated by the wish to have everything in perfect formation before he returns to work. As a consequence, he remains angry, frustrated, inactive, and unoccupied.

Environmental advocacy is often particularly important for those who have impulsive and dissocial personalities. Another patient with whom we have been involved for nearly 20 years has such a short attention span that he could be accurately diagnosed as having ADHD. He is intelligent and quick to learn, but he so quickly tires of any repetitive work that he never lasts for more than a few days. All the time, he is looking for a quick fix, and it has been impossible to train him to a sufficient extent for him to hold down the type of job he would be quite capable of carrying out. But we have not excluded him from occupational activity. One of the amazing benefits of living in the United Kingdom is that there are dozens of charities that have unlimited patience and amazing flexibility in what they can offer people who come for help. One place that I have found to be especially helpful is a barge floating on the River Thames that takes patients with chronic psychiatric disorders who have often been rejected elsewhere. There is no attempt to give them any form of standard psychological therapy; instead, they are given the option of a large range of woodcarving activities covering a wide range of skills but beginning with carving that everyone is capable of achieving. People who attend the barge know the times of opening and closing, but they can come at any time during these periods and are welcomed. Some who have been unemployed for years and have very few human contacts find coming to the barge a very fruitful social experience and have been attending for years. There is no limit on the period of attendance, and the standard leaving statement 'You have finished your course of treatment' does not apply. The rehabilitation barge is an excellent example of a service adapting to the needs of personality-disordered people and the complementary action of people adapting to the barge. It is a very harmonious relationship. We have not yet succeeded in getting my highly impulsive patient to engage fully with the barge but have not stopped trying. (See the details of the barge, Cathja, in the acknowledgment section of this book.)

Some of the more difficult problems in finding a way forward to solve environmental needs are ones in which the person is perceived by everybody as needing a change of environment, but this is resisted by the person concerned. Perhaps the most common example of this is elderly people needing support who are still living in the accommodation where they have spent most of their lives. Often, this accommodation is highly unsuitable and sometimes dangerous, but change to a different accommodation is strongly resisted. It is in these situations that a strong environmental advocate is needed. Nidotherapists always listen very carefully to people's wishes and try as much as possible to agree to them. But in these situations, it is very difficult to support the patient if they really are in a perilous situation by continuing to stay where they are.

Those with detached and anankastic personality patterns are much more likely to be resistive to change in such circumstances. I cannot pretend that we have solved this particular problem, but the range of strategies we have tried to use to get approval for appropriate changes to be made include test trials in different environments; creating a checklist of all the necessary requirements that would need to be present in the new setting; getting assessments from organisations such as the fire service, social services, and environmental agencies about the risks of continuing to live in the old environment; and offers to stay in the new environment once the transfer has been made. But with all these possible solutions, it is important not to resort to threats in order to force the issue.

Phase 4. Monitoring the nidopathway

This last phase of nidotherapy has so much variability that it is difficult to formulate it systematically. If the task is fairly straightforward—e.g., please enable my discharge from hospital (the most common request of the Victorian mental hospital patient)—it may be regarded as complete as soon as the patient has been placed elsewhere. But this only applies when others are involved and can take on other roles in management. If the nidotherapist is working in a system which is not supporting the decisions made in treatment, then it may be necessary for the therapist to remain in contact for many months to get all the environmental changes completed. It is not possible to give firm advice here, but in some cases, we have had to remain in contact with patients for many years because our service is regarded as a lifeline.

Often there are concerns expressed, usually by those who do not quite understand the purpose of nidotherapy, that people will become overdependent on their therapist, and the relationship then gets very complicated. But this is very rarely happens. If the nidotherapist is regarded as an environmental aide who understands the needs of the person but is not emotionally close to them, then abnormal dependence does not arise. But of course we have to recognise that many people with personality problems are highly dependent, and this has to be acknowledged in choosing the environmental changes. If it is made absolutely clear from the beginning that dependence on the therapist is not anything more than a temporary manoeuvre in the course of treatment, then long-term problems do not arise.

This does not mean that nidotherapy is free of risks, especially with those who have personality problems of any severity. Here is an example of a very complex problem that we think we solved by nidotherapy but which also led to attendant problems.

Case example: the inveterate hoarder with a literary bent

Describing the different phases of nidotherapy is necessary but is not intellectually challenging. There is no central concept requiring great depth of thought, and a great many of the suggestions made in the different phases of treatment could be regarded as simple common sense. This is one of the reasons we think that all therapists ought to have knowledge of nidotherapy as an extra arm in their treatment armamentarium, to be called on when necessary but not to dominate practice. But in the case I am about to describe, it did unfortunately dominate my practice for several months and led to me moving my clinical work to a different area.

Henry (not his real name) was a man who lived in a house on the bottom floor of a large housing estate in central London. He suffered from a very severe personality disorder in which the detached and anankastic domains were both very prominent. He had never had any meaningful relationships except with his family, and even these had led to considerable suffering. This included breaking his mother's arm in an argument and having a very fraught relationship with his sister, who did her best to try and maintain his links with society with stoic determination. He had a degree in English and was highly intelligent but because of his personality difficulties had never worked for more than a few months and had not worked in the 15 years before we saw him as a patient. The reason he was referred was that he suffered from a disorder called hoarding disorder, a condition that did not officially exist when our team was first seeing him.

It is now a formal diagnosis in ICD-11 and is defined as

repetitive urges or behaviours related to amassing items, which may be passive (e.g. accumulation of incoming flyers or mail) or active (e.g. excessive acquisition of free, purchased or stolen items); and

- difficulty discarding possessions due to a perceived need to save items, and distress associated with discarding them.
- The symptoms result in significant distress or significant impairment in personal, family, social, educational, occupational or other important areas of functioning.

(World Health Organisation, 2024, p. 322)

There is wide variation in hoarding behaviour, and in Henry's case, he was right at the most severe end of the spectrum. Some who hoard acknowledge that many of the items they save are without value and unlikely to be of future use and admit that any distress they feel when discarding items is not rational. But at the other extreme are people like Henry, who are convinced that their beliefs and their need to hoard are perfectly rational, and sometimes the strength of these can be considered to be delusional because of their intensity of conviction.

The consequence of hoarding is that people accumulate vast amounts of unnecessary items in their living quarters, and this sometimes assumes such proportions that the cubic capacity of vacant space is usually found only high up near the ceiling—every other gap is filled. It takes a very strong personality to work with hoarders successfully; Elaine Birchall and Suzanne Cronkwright describe the qualities you need to do it extremely well (Birchall & Cronkwright, 2019). But Henry had strong reasons for his hoarding behaviour. He was an eco-warrior. (This was in 1999, before most people started getting concerned about climate change.) He hated all forms of plastic covering and would only eat food when he could cook it 'naked'. He also believed that virtually every object should be recycled rather than relegated to a rubbish tip. The fact that he was on the ground floor of a large council block was unfortunate because when his neighbours left wardrobes, chairs, and similar items of furniture out for waste collection, Henry anticipated their arrival and moved all these objects into his flat.

Because there were so little space in the flat, Henry was unable to do any cooking, and most of the food he ate was raw. We could never understand why he did not become ill because he tended to leave his food in the open for days until it started to rot. 'It always tastes sweeter then', he argued.

But Henry was not only a hoarder; he had prolonged periods of depression. Even though he preferred being on his own, he liked talking to people, an activity which he took literally as he did virtually all the talking. He became particularly attached to a female social worker, and when she had to move to a different area, he made out that she had left voluntarily because she was so fed up meeting with him. He loved saying that he was the unhappiest person in the world, but he could not make any comparisons; he did not know anybody apart from his professional visitors.

I got into the habit of seeing him at the same time each week—Henry always wanted to know at what time you were visiting—and I enjoyed sparring with him over the English language. He argued that all the adjectives and adverbs that began with the prefix 'un' applied to him as they described his miserable state, but when I said his command of the language was unbeatable, he found it difficult to do it down.

People with hoarding disorder can live for years without interruption, but this becomes more difficult if they live in a flat in a council block. Over the course of time, Henry's flat became more and more offensive to neighbours as the smell of his rotting food and the constellation of flies throughout the flat attracted the attention of many. Henry claimed that his hygiene and cooking arrangements were no concern of others, but the pressure to change matters continued to increase. It was felt that he had to be committed to hospital for the sake of his health and that of others, and consideration was given to a rarely used section of the mental health act concerned with public health and safety.

In the end, he was admitted under the conventional section to our inpatient unit. Westminster City Council agreed to clear out the flat, and this was done smartly, to the satisfaction of Henry's neighbours. But the council was also contracted to refurbish the flat, and this seemed to have no time scale. Henry remained in hospital, rather dissatisfied at the loss of all his belongings, and his admission was not serving any useful purpose.

He continued to agitate for his discharge, and our clinical team had to agree with him. He also had clear ideas about how he wanted to redecorate his flat, and these were quite different from the expectations of Westminster City Council.

It was at this point that nidotherapy and Henry's wishes joined together with my own personality deviation. I felt it was quite inappropriate to keep Henry in hospital at the cost of nearly £1000 per day with no immediate prospect of discharge. Both the impulsive and obsessional components of my personality took over. I could not justify unnecessary state expenditure for someone who did not need to be in hospital, and I had a solution to his redecorating that was entirely to Henry's satisfaction. So I barged ahead.

The solution involved redecorating Henry's flat to his own specifications. These were not normal expectations. He wanted his walls painted in magnolia and his doors in grey and had specific requirements for all his other rooms. It did not require much persuading for our clinical team to agree to carry out the decorations so Henry could be discharged with a minimum of furniture. Unfortunately, although the clinical team agreed, the attendant social services involved with Henry were against this idea, and when it was implemented, a formal complaint was made to the Trust about Professor Tyrer's malpractice. But by the time the complaint was investigated, Henry had already been discharged to his new purpose-decorated flat and was very satisfied with this.

But the formal complaint went through a full investigation by the chief nursing officer, and in the final verdict, I was criticised strongly for initiating the plan to decorate Henry's flat. The verdict included the interesting statement, 'Peter Tyrer always likes to do the best for his patients but does not always go about it in the right way'. Now, more than 20 years later, I am still not sure whether I would or should have acted differently if presented with the same dilemma again. I was following all the ten principles of nidotherapy—All people have the capacity to improve their lives when placed in the right environment (Henry was quite clear what the 'right environment' was); everyone should have the chance to test themselves in environments of their own choosing (Henry supervised the decorating); when people become distressed without apparent reason, the cause can often be found in the immediate environment (Henry was very distressed with the inpatient hospital environment); a person's environment includes not only place but also other people and self (Henry was a detached loner; he found many people very difficult to tolerate); seeing the world through another's eyes gives a better perspective than your eyes alone (Henry's vision of a good flat was very different from that of Westminster City Council); what someone else thinks is the best environment for a person isn't necessarily so (three resounding cheers from Henry for that); all people, no matter how disabled or handicapped, have strengths that can be fostered (Henry was odd but determined; he always made his opinions very clear); a person's environment should never be regarded as impossible to change (we followed this to the letter); every environmental change involves some risk, but this is not a reason to avoid it (we could have had accidents with nurses falling off ladders while painting the ceilings, Westminster City Council blocking entry to Henry's flat, Peter Tyrer being sacked from his position, but these were not reasons for passive behaviour); and mutual collaboration is required to change environments for the better (we were certainly mutual in the joint planning of our enterprise).

I was also acting in a cost-effective way as our team decorating saved Westminster City Council a considerable sum (we paid for it ourselves), and his early discharge saved the NHS at least £50,000 as there was no clear date to redecorate his flat by the time he left hospital. Was all this worth an expensive internal inquiry and a critical report? Should I have been less confrontational and tried to get agreement before decorating the flat, and was my personality getting in the way of a better resolution? Perhaps I and the team should have just stomached the system with a grimace and grumbled only to our colleagues without doing anything more? I would like to feel that in the future the principles of nidotherapy might be followed by all services (see Chapter 15) so this type of practice could be embraced rather than challenged but will leave this to the reader to decide. Henry, a short time later, was relocated to a support hostel as his block of flats, overlooking Paddington Basin, was one of the most salubrious pieces of real estate in the area. It was razed to the ground and replaced by a 12-storey glass and shining white edifice in which I am sure magnolia walls are in short supply. But Henry was not forgotten; he was one the fictional heroes of a book in which the Earth was saved from extinction by the deflection of an asteroid (Tyrer, 2020)—the ultimate success of the eco-warrior.

Henry's account represents the extremes of nidotherapy. Those with severe personality disorder, almost systematically without ever realising it. close down all the environmental options that might otherwise be available to them, and opening up each of them again requires a tremendous amount of effort that some would say is not worthwhile.

My view is that the impressions created by the more severe personality disorders have promoted stigma and wrongly influenced all the negative attitudes about the subject, which are only gradually being changed in society—Gwen Adshead's Reith Lectures (2024) helping greatly in this respect.

THE IMPORTANCE OF NIDOTHERAPY WHEN EVERYBODY ELSE HAS
REJECTED INTERVENTION FOR THOSE WITH PERSONALITY DISORDERS

Henry's case illustrates the laid-back indifference that many practitioners feel when presented with people who have the most intractable personality disorders. 'Why are you bothering, Peter?' I used to be asked. 'You're wasting your time with these people; there are many more who want your help and would respond to it. Go and see them instead'.

My answer is the same as that inscribed on the Wedgwood anti-slavery medallion—a kneeling black man in chains with his hands raised to the heavens, who says 'Am I not a man and a brother?' I cannot make the trite statement 'Some of my best friends have severe personality disorder', but I can say 'Those with severe personality disorder can have friends who care'.

The prejudiced attitudes started early and always seem to have been attracted to the severe end of the spectrum. One hundred seventy-two years ago, Morel, a French physician, divided patient into six groups, one of which was equivalent to personality disorders, which he claimed were determined by heredity and who 'in consequence of their hereditary taint, display their insanity in actions rather than words—in eccentricities, incoherence, irregularity and often extreme immorality of conduct' (Morel, 1852).

This unimpressive curriculum vitae was added to by the famous English psychiatrist Henry Maudsley, who also specially selected those who possessed all the features of dissociality by describing them as

> inherently vicious, instinctive liars and thieves, stealing and deceiving with a cunning and a skill which could never be acquired; they display no trace of affection for their parents, or of feelings for others; the only care they evince is to contrive the means of indulging their passions and vicious propensities.
>
> (Maudsley, 1868, p. 329)

This was developed further. As mentioned earlier, Koch, in Germany, (1891) greatly emphasised this notion of hereditary untreatability by suggesting that all those with personality disorder were constitutionally inferior because of degeneration of their nervous systems.

After reading this background history, it is not at all surprising that personality disturbance has continued to attract such prejudice and stigma, added to by the notion of untreatability that has put it in the same bracket as leprosy before there was any treatment available. Quite simply, people is this group were regarded as highly unpleasant, untreatable people who were damned by their constitutions and heredity to become permanent outlaws from respectable society.

Attempts to change this perception have only been partly successful. Past history takes years to correct, and, despite a tremendous effort to turn this around in recent years, most people still have an aversion to the whole concept. As Ferguson and I commented in 2000,

> It belongs to psychiatry and yet is strangely apart, and at various times we have tried to dismiss it from our professional consciousness. It is a concept like body odour, indubitably affected by constitution and environment, a source of distress to both sufferer and society, yet imbued with ideas of degeneracy and inferiority so that its possession is also a personal criticism.
>
> (Ferguson & Tyrer, 2000)

Another reason given to me for not bothering to try and help people with many personality problems is that most people with these disorders do not ask for help and will not thank you for attempting to provide it. This is partly a consequence of their inability to recognise that they have any kind of problem, partly a feeling of annoyance that people are trying to prevent them from living the lives they want to lead, and partly because they are proud to be the way they are and highly protective of their inner beings. The last of these wishes everybody would share but most of us forget the other two. The treatment-resistant (Type R) personalities (Tyrer et al., 2003) are more than twice the number as the Type S treatment-seeking personalities who dominate the media air waves.

The wish to avoid treatment explains why all the many treatments described in Chapter 4 are for the dubious disorder called borderline or emotional instability; the others reject any attempts to interfere with their personalities with indifference or scorn. 'I am what I am; how dare you try and change me'.

The advantage of nidotherapy in this context is crystal clear. 'We are not trying to change you', I say repeatedly. ' We are just trying to change your environment so that you fit in better'. Once this message has sunk home, there is no difficulty in engaging with options for change. The only problem that all nidotherapists encounter in those with severe personality disorder is that the number of environmental options in this group is sometimes vanishingly small.

When people ask me, 'How can nidotherapy help people if you do not classify it as a treatment?' I respond, 'Adaptation to the environment may be a manouevre, a strategy, an approach, a selected intervention, a scheme, a ploy, or a plan, but no matter what you call it, the outcome is intended to be positive for mental health'.

This explains a paradox. If most people retain their personality status over time, as all the evidence suggests they do (Costa et al., 2019), why does personality disorder appear to change, particularly if you argue that the personality spectrum includes all? The answer is 'adaptation'. If the person moves into an environment that makes a more adaptive fit, then the disorder disappears, even though the basic personality remains the same. A mistake that may sometimes be made is for therapists to concentrate on changing a specific trait or characteristic in a personality. It may seem to work in the short term, but it will not last unless it coincides with environmental change. Hard-working therapists have been trying to do this for years with the polyglot language of borderline without success.

Many years ago, I suggested a way of explaining personality disorder that renamed it more accurately. I suggested the term 'personality diathesis'. This was summarised thus:

> [T]he diathesis, or vulnerability, model identifies an innate tendency to
> develop other disorders more frequently,
> and both to increase their intensity and
> frequency of recurrence. Thus, those with abnormal
> personalities can be seen as having an
> Achilles' heel that allows the individual to
> function normally in most circumstances but
> when faced with certain situations becomes activated
> and precipitates problems.
>
> (Tyrer, 2007, p. 1522)

This terminology explains why personality disorders are not cured in the medical sense but also not persistently manifest; they come and go depending on environmental stimuli of all kinds. Only a full understanding of nidotherapy can help predict the course of someone with a personality problem.

Because the basic building blocks of nidotherapy involve an understanding of the links between person and environment, it requires a different type of therapist from most others. As noted, a key element is to get inside the head and understand the thinking of the person you are trying to help. This may take the therapist into new territory at times, but if the principles of nidotherapy are remembered, they remain as useful anchors.

So who could be able to call themselves a nidotherapist? Quite a few. If a person is released from prison by an executive order, this is not nidotherapy, but if the release is pre-planned and the prisoner leaves to a successful coordinated rehabilitation setting, this is a form of nidotherapy. We also know this is successful. In the first trial of nidotherapy (Ranger et al., 2009), patients allocated randomly to nidotherapy had much more structured and careful discharge plans than others in the second randomised group, so the placements chosen for them were not just made in a hurry;

they were planned so they fitted, as much as possible, the wishes and needs of the people who were going to live in them. As a consequence, the incidence of relapse and readmission was much less than in the group who did not receive this extra matching of person to environment. They were more likely to fail and to be readmitted. Not surprisingly, the nidotherapy intervention was more cost effective. The planning of discharge consisted of a careful review of what each patient wanted and what was available. It was an important task but not one that required high-powered clinical skills.

One of the difficulties in assessing the impact of interventions for personality disorder is the lack of the agreed outcomes that constitute success (Tyrer & Sharp, 2023). What is more important, an ability to live independently, an improvement in social networks, a lessening of hostility towards others, greater self-sufficiency, occupational success, or an increase in the positive emotions of contentment and goodwill? There is no agreement on this matter, but the strongest claim can be made for overall improvement in social function as the prime index of success (Tyrer et al., 2021).

The reasoning behind this fits in very well with nidotherapy, as better social function indicates successful adaptation (Tyrer et al., 2021), and once a positive change in social functioning is achieved, all the other elements of successful treatment tend to follow suit. Using the old criteria of DSM and ICD, the personality disorder may stick, but with the ICD-11 system, there will be a bonfire of change (Yang et al., 2022).

So if nidotherapy is so valuable, you may ask, why can I not be trained in it using a health technology training module like MBT, CBT, TFT, SFT, and all the other three-letter acronyms that litter our professional lives? The reason for this is simple. If the intention in treatment is to listen carefully to people, find out their many needs and aspirations, and then advise or facilitate their making appropriate changes, then you cannot plan *in advance* exactly what you are going to do. You can adopt a set of strategies, as indeed is the case with nidotherapy in following assessment of the person with an environmental analysis and planned timetable, but it is just not possible to plan everything at the outset. It is also often not possible to determine how long a nidotherapy intervention will take; it can vary from a few days to a few years.

The absence of a repeatable module with standard instructions has one major handicap. It makes it much more difficult to carry out evaluative research studies and also to train investigators in the appropriate methodology. We have sometimes been criticised for not carrying out more research trials in nidotherapy, but they are not easy to mount. The two trials we were able to complete (Ranger et al., 2009; Tyrer et al., 2017) did involve specific forms of nidotherapy, the sensitive placement of patients with severe mental illness and personality problems after discharge from hospital, and the management of challenging behaviour in those with intellectual disability in care homes. These involved focused, not general nidotherapy and were appropriate for these populations only.

But this does not mean you cannot be trained in nidotherapy. Apart from books such as this one and others (Akerman et al., 2018; Tyrer, 2009, 2018; Tyrer & Tyrer, 2018), there is a CPD training module on nidotherapy at the Royal College of Psychiatrists; an annual workshop and training programme at the Nidotherapy Advice and Training Centre at Cotham, Nottinghamshire; and a website (www.nidotherapy.co.uk) that keeps all up to date.

References

Akerman G, Needs A, & Bainbridge C (eds) (2018). *Transforming Environments and Rehabilitation: A Guide for Practitioners in Forensic Settings and Criminal Justice*. Abingdon: Routledge.

Birchall E & Cronkwright S (2019). *Conquer the Clutter: Strategies to Identify, Manage, and Overcome Hoarding*. Johns Hopkins University Press.

Costa PT Jr, McCrae RR, & Löckenhoff CE (2019). Personality across the life span. *Annual Review of Psychology*, 70, 423–448.

Ferguson B & Tyrer P (2000). History of the concept of personality disorder. In: *Personality Disorders: Diagnosis, Management and Course* (2nd edition, p. 11) Oxford; Boston: Butterworth Heinemann.

Goodman R (1997). The Strengths and Difficulties Questionnaire: a research note. *Journal of Child Psychology and Psychiatry*, 38, 581–586.

Koch J (1891–3). *Die psychopathischen Minderwertigkeiten* (3 vols.). Ravensburg: Maier.

Maudsley H (1868). *A Physiology and Pathology of Mind* (2nd edition). Macmillan.

Morel BA (1852). *Traité Theorique et Pratique des Maladies*. Baillière.

Ranger M, Tyrer P, Miloseska K, Fourie H, Khaleel I, North B, et al. (2009). Cost-effectiveness of nidotherapy for comorbid personality disorder and severe mental illness: randomized controlled trial. *Epidemiologia e Psichiatria Sociale*, 18, 128–136.

Tribe RH, Freeman AM, Livingstone S, Stott JCH, & Pilling S (2019). Open dialogue in the UK: qualitative study. *BJPsych Open*, 5, e49.

Tyrer P (2002). Nidotherapy: a new approach to the treatment of personality disorder. *Acta Psychiatrica Scandinavica*, 105, 469–471.

Tyrer P (2007). Personality diatheses: a superior description than disorder. *Psychological Medicine*, 37, 1521–1525.

Tyrer P (2009). *Nidotherapy: Harmonising the Environment with the Patient*. London: RCPsych Press.

Tyrer P (2018). *Taming the Beast Within: Shredding the Stereotypes of Personality Disorder*. London: Sheldon Press.

Tyrer P (2020). *Millie & Oscar Go Loco*. Kibworth: The Book Guild Ltd.

Tyrer P, Mitchard S, Methuen C, & Ranger M (2003). Treatment-rejecting and treatment-seeking personality disorders: Type R and Type S. *Journal of Personality Disorders*, 17, 265–270.

Tyrer P & Sharp C (2023). Establishing efficacy and effectiveness in the treatment of personality disorders. *Personality and Mental Health*, 17, 295–299.

Tyrer P, Tarabi SA, Bassett P, Liedtka N, Hall R, Nagar J, et al. (2017). Nidotherapy compared with enhanced care programme approach training for adults with aggressive challenging behaviour and intellectual disability (NIDABID): cluster-randomised controlled trial. *Journal of Intellectual Disability Research*, 61, 521–531.

Tyrer P & Tyrer H (2018). *Nidotherapy: Harmonising the Environment with the Patient* (2nd edition). Cambridge: Cambridge University Press.

Tyrer P, Yang M, Tyrer H, & Crawford M (2021). Is social function a good proxy measure of personality disorder? *Personality and Mental Health*, 15, 261–272.

World Health Organisation (2024). *Clinical Descriptions and Diagnostic Requirements for ICD-11 Mental, Behavioural and Neurodevelopmental Disorders*. Geneva.

Yang M, Tyrer P, & Tyrer H (2022). The recording of personality strengths: an analysis of the impact of positive personality features on the long-term outcome of common mental disorders. *Personality and Mental Health*, 16, 120–129.

Chapter 8

Adapting to personality difficulty

Personality difficulty is the easiest form of personality disturbance to adapt to practice, but it deserves a chapter on its own as it is a good marker for other, more complex adaptive needs. This is because personality difficulty, by its definition, only manifests itself in certain situations. This allows plans for dealing with these situations to be made in advance. The situations creating the difficulty vary but are likely to occur fairly frequently to be manifest as personality difficulty as, if they are rare, the personality problems will only be shown to a very few people. In this chapter, the different ways in which personality difficulty can be expressed are described and methods of adapting to them examined with examples. The examples are based on my clinical experience but have been disguised to avoid identification of any particular individual.

The definition of personality difficulty in ICD-11 is:

Box 8.1 The formal definition of personality difficulty in ICD-11

Personality difficulty is characterized by longstanding difficulties (e.g. at least 2 years) in the individual's way of experiencing and thinking about the self, others and the world. In contrast to personality disorder, personality difficulty is manifested in cognitive and emotional experience and expression only intermittently (e.g. during times of stress) or at low intensity. Personality difficulty is typically associated with some problems in functioning but these are insufficiently severe to cause notable disruption in social occupational and interpersonal relationships or may be limited to specific relationships or situations.

(World Health Organisation, 2024, p. 559)

DOI: 10.4324/9781003560630-8

The nature of personality difficulty can be further described using the five trait domain specifiers mentioned previously—negative affectivity, detachment, dissociality, disinhibition, and anankastia.

Some people do not like the idea of this group being in the classification of personality disorder and have accused the ICD-11 group of 'medicalising' the whole population with an offensive label of stigma. The precise opposite is true. Because epidemiological studies have found that sub-threshold personality problems, not severe enough to be called personality disorder, are more common than any other group on the personality spectrum, this confirms the merits of a diagnostic system comprising a spectrum of personality. As most of us therefore show some evidence of disorder, we can say with a touch of pride, 'Almost all of us have disturbed personalities; let us rejoice and revel in our diversity and forget all about stigma'.

We have not yet reached the point when a politician can respond in a debate in the House of Commons by saying, 'I apologise to the honourable member for the strength of my language. I was allowing my personality difficulty to get the better of me'. But we may not be far off once the importance of this area of pathology becomes recognised.

Because personality difficulty has only just been given approval as what could be called, rather clumsily, a subsyndromal form of personality dysfunction, it is not known how it should best be managed and to what extent mental health professionals should be involved in recognising it. I give examples of five people, each showing personality difficulty in a different domain, to show how it can be changed successfully.

Example 1. Personality difficulty in the negative emotional domain

Stanley was 56, and, after being made redundant from his job at the age of 55, he decided not to work again. He had never liked his job working as an overlocking machine assistant in a clothing factory where he was with a large number of women, among whom he felt intimidated. He felt anxious and inadequate amongst them, had very little conversation, and often got into arguments over silly matters. He often dwelt on these troubles and had difficulty sleeping. After he retired, he met a friend in a pub one evening and was told about a vacancy at the local garden allotments. Stanley was persuaded to visit and decided to take up the vacant allotment. He was a competent gardener, learnt quickly, and was a highly successful grower. He became much more confident, lost his anxiety, slept soundly, and generated many new friends. Shortly afterward, he became the secretary of the allotment group, a position in which he felt very proud. For the first time in his life, he felt all his talents were being used.

It is easy to see why this transformation occurred. Stanley was in the wrong working environment for most of his working life. Being naturally anxious and mildly fearful, he had drifted into his job without ever seeking it, had never fitted in, and had not had the courage or opportunity to change. Redundancy, often thought of as a loss, gave him the chance for a rethink, and in his new environment, he found a perfect environmental fit.

Example 2. Personality difficulty in the detached domain

Frank was an only child, and his parents hoped that when he went to school, he would make many new friends. But he did not. He remained isolated and was bullied frequently, often coming home in tears. He was slow to learn in many subjects, and it was only when he was a little older that it was noted he was gifted in mathematics. He obtained a place at university and was very successful there in examinations but failed to make any new relationships there. His family was afraid he might finish up on the sidelines of life, but after a meeting with one of the senior professors at the university, they were told, 'Frank is an excellent mathematician, and he could forge an excellent career in statistics. It matters not a jot that he is a bit isolated; many mathematicians are. I will look out some possible options for him; he will certainly not be forgotten'.

Subsequently, Frank became a research fellow at a highly respected research unit, published many breakthrough papers, and achieved high regard from colleagues. He remained detached and lived alone but did not have any regrets about what to others would be regarded as an unsatisfactory lifestyle.

Example 3. Personality difficulty in the impulsive domain

Beryl was a hard-working nursery nurse who was very popular with all her staff. She never had a great deal of money and had a tendency to spend a little unwisely on impulse. After she had to spend more than usual on nursery care for her daughter, she took to gambling online to try and make up the difference. At first she was successful, and this encouraged her to gamble more, but then she started getting into serious financial difficulty. She also put on weight and stopped exercising. After getting advice from her GP about exercise, she decided to take up jogging whenever she was bored and enticed by gambling again and became very keen on getting a jogging index, a calculation first described by a physicist called Harold Jeffreys many years ago. Harold called his the bicycle index, which indicated the number of times he had cycled a certain distance. So when he raised his bicycle index to 20, this indicated that he had cycled 20 miles on 20 occasions. Beryl was determined to get her jogging index up to five and persuaded—if that is the right word—her husband to pay her a reward when she had jogged for five miles on five occasions. She steadily increased her jogging index, and the excitement of getting a reward each time satisfied her gambling instincts, made her fitter, and solved her financial problems.

Example 4. Personality difficulty in the dissocial domain

Derek was a tearaway at school, always cheeking the teachers and playing truant, getting involved in fights, and eventually being expelled. His parents recognised that he had abilities, but he was so restricted by authority and always had to fight against it. Partly related to worry about Derek, but also because they saw better opportunities abroad, the family decided to emigrate to Australia. They decided not to stay in the urban areas and carved out a new life for themselves in the bush. Derek was so much happier with his new freedom and blossomed, eventually going to agricultural college and becoming a farmer. Always willing to try new approaches, even if they were a bit risky, he took on a farm in a very sparsely populated rural area. He had cattle spread over hundreds of acres and found it very difficult to protect and herd them. He worked out that the best way of controlling their movements was to supervise herding from the air. He learnt how to fly helicopters and before long was able to herd them to the best pastures and also protect them from dangerous terrain. He became highly successful and was praised as a pioneer of this new form of farming.

Example 5. Personality difficulty in the anankastic domain

Julie was always keen on computers at school and was very pleased when she was able to get a job as a web designer. She worked with a small team and quickly impressed them by the speed with which she picked up new techniques. Before long she became the senior member of the team. It was at this point that others noticed things were going wrong. The other members of the team, especially new appointees, were taking more time off sick and complained of stress at work. A senior member of the company was asked to investigate. He quickly found out that Julie was not only doing her own job but interfering with the work of all the others, as she was so determined to make sure that everything was done to her own high standards. This interference had caused much upset.

Julie was interviewed and agreed that she had been supervising all her colleagues, even though this was not in her job description. She apologised through tears for letting the company down. She was reassured that all could be put right, and a change in her work was agreed. She was taken off her job on the team and given the task of working on her own in developing new web technologies. Freed from the need to supervise others, Julie thrived, and all the difficulties with the other staff evaporated away.

The problems of each of the five people described here were not ones that the average professional in practice would recognise to be clinically significant. Most of the time, they would hardly be recognised at all as the problems created would be too minor to ever lead to professional advice. It will also be noticed that the people who changed the environment of each of these people—a pub friend, a mathematics professor, a GP (seeing her for weight problems), a concerned family, and a company executive—were not in any way professionals in mental health. But they were nonetheless acting as nidotherapists by recognising a misfit between the person and the environment that could be solved by adapting the personality to a different environment.

The examples also need to be qualified. They describe each example as though the person's personality was dominated by a single domain trait. In practice, any number of domain traits can be present in a person and so influence behaviour. But they do show that the principles of adaptation aided by nidotherapy are successful in compensating for personality difficulty and often convert what was previously a difficulty into an asset. This should be treasured.

Reference

World Health Organisation (2024). *Clinical Descriptions and Diagnostic Requirements for ICD-11 Mental, Behavioural and Neurodevelopmental Disorders.* WHO: Geneva.

Chapter 9

Adapting to negative affectivity

Negative affectivity is a complex polysyllable that covers the full range of emotions. Together these make up the range of moods, a wide span from depression and anger to anxiety, fear, and shame.

This includes many aspects of the better known adjective, borderline, and many may prefer this term in spite of the heavy criticism I have directed at it elsewhere in this book. But I will not be discussing the issue of borderline or emotional dysregulation in this chapter; it has already been dissected in Chapter 4. In making the distinction between emotional dysregulation and negative affectivity, which many people join together wrongly, the important difference is that negative affectivity is a long-standing personality trait whereas emotional dysregulation is episodic, often temporary, and not a personality domain.

It is also useful to separate the forms in which negative emotions are shown: those that are directed outwards (externalizing), such as hostility, paranoia, anger, and scorn, all of which have a great impact on others, and those directed inwards (internalizing), such as guilt, depression, self-criticism, and anxiety, which are much less prominent and often remain hidden.

These feelings may change greatly from day to day and even in the course of conversation with others. The emotions often seem to take over every part of the person's function and prevent any rational discussion.

In adapting this domain to become more helpful, I summarise again three of the characteristics of each domain.

Stage 1: Identify negative affectivity and the environments in which it most manifest

External negative affectivity

It is relatively easy to identify the environments which illustrate the external aspects of negative affectivity; they are all concerned in interactions

DOI: 10.4324/9781003560630-9

with people. A person with only a cat for company stranded on a desert island at first might have a few negative interactions with the cat—'come down from that coconut palm immediately'—but, as cats do not respond in kind, harmony would soon be restored. The people who appear to create most emotional turmoil are usually identified without any difficulty, and the ones who are central to bad experiences are often those whom it is impossible to avoid.

Internal negative affectivity

Many fail to identify inner emotional turmoil unless they are good observers, and even then, there is an element of guesswork and puzzlement. In Jane Austen's novel *Sense and Sensibility*, the two sisters, Marianne and Elinor, differ greatly in their emotional expression, with Marianne's feelings bursting out uncontrollably while those of her sister are snuffed and suppressed. Jane Austen hits the affectivity nail on the head precisely when the two sisters decide they have nothing to say to each other as one conceals nothing and the other communicates nothing. The uncommunicating person, overwhelmed with internal negative affectivity, has a library of content waiting to be delivered, but the library is seldom open to visitors, and the books just get moved around from shelf to shelf.

So the person with this kind of internal turmoil spends hours mulling over and ruminating about how they should react to the people they both hate and love, in what way they should change, and how they should interpret what others are saying and rehearsing forthcoming events in a way that will never come to pass. In writing about nidotherapy, I have referred to the Prufrock syndrome (Tyrer, 2009), named after the eponymous centre-piece of TS Eliot's famous poem *The Love Song of J. Alfred Prufrock*. The parody is in the title, as the poem shows that poor Alfred has no love in his life. He is just rocked by doubt in his internal negative world as he sits and watches others:

> *Time for you and time for me,*
> *And time yet for a hundred indecisions,*
> *And for a hundred visions and revisions,*
> *Before the taking of a toast and tea.*

But he doesn't make decisions; he just watches others and ruminates:

> *For I have known them all already, known them all:*
> *Have known the evenings, mornings, afternoons,*
> *I have measured out my life with coffee spoons;*

I know the voices dying with a dying fall
Beneath the music from a farther room.
So how should I presume?

The Prufrock syndrome is the antithesis of action: a continual mulling over that has no end and leads to no decisions.

These types of environment are easily identifiable. The best form of immediate adaptation for both of them is avoidance, but this is much easier to achieve with external negative affectivity. Those preoccupied with the internal form can easily develop a continuous preoccupation of worry. Often this extends to health, and this can become such a concern it binds in the whole personality to such an extent that hypochondriasis becomes a personality disorder in its own right (Tyrer et al., 1990). Once established, it can persist for many years (Tyrer et al., 1999).

Boswell's biography of the polymath Samuel Johnson is an account by one hypochondriacal personality of another and describes over and over the relapsing nature of the condition, together with its association with depression.

Madmen are all sensual in the lower stages of distemper. They are eager for gratification to soothe their minds, and divert their attention from the misery they suffer; but when they grow very ill, pleasure is too weak for them, and they seek for pain.

(Boswell, September 20, 1791, p. 311)

'When I survey my past life, I discover nothing but a barren waste of time, with some disorders of body, and disturbances of the mind very near to madness' (Boswell, 1791, p. 296). Not long before Johnson's death, '[H]e suffered a very severe return of the hypochondriac disorder, which was ever lurking about him. He was so ill, as, notwithstanding his remarkable love of company, to be entirely averse to society, the most fatal symptom of that malady' (p. 114). 'He was afflicted by a bodily disease, which made him often restless and fretful, and with a constitutional melancholy, the clouds of which darkened the brightness of his fancy' (p. 500).

Those who suffer the fearful ruminations of hypochondriacal negative affectivity should have our sympathy; it takes hard work to drive them away.

Stage 2: Test out the environments that best compensate for or nullify negative affectivity

For external negative affectivity, avoidance can be practised readily by identifying all the people who add to feelings of anger and annoyance and making as little contact with them as possible. For those who cannot be avoided as contact is necessary for any reason, a tone of smiling tolerance needs to be generated, a tone that is obviously artificial but is not too difficult after a little practice. If your life course involves such negative interactions and is constantly being disrupted by anxiety and distress, you need to think carefully about changing it drastically. There are very many ways in which altering your activities in a planned way leaves you in greater control of your destiny. A useful concept here is called locus of control (Rotter, 1990). Those with an internal locus of control place themselves in environments where they are able to influence strongly their own actions, people, and events, whereas those with an external locus of control are in environments where they are tossed about by fate and chance and have very little say in what happens.

The research evidence suggests those with an external locus of control (LOC) are more likely than others to experience negative affective symptoms over time. In one seven-year study, those with an external LOC predicted higher anxiety and depression severity but did not influence the incidence of positive and negative life events (Hovenkamp-Hermelink et al., 2019). I have argued in other parts of this book that successful nidotherapy would have influenced life events more.

So, consider: if your interactions are dominated by an external locus of control, do you need to re-evaluate your priorities? Of course, many are forced by circumstance to be buffeted by influences that they can do little to alter, but none of us are completely dominated by external events. 'How can I bring back control of my life?' is a question that should be asked, and it cannot be answered by the blanket 'It is not possible', unless you are in an imprisoned closed environment like Alexei Navalny.

But even in the prison of complete external locus of control, you can still come to terms with negative affectivity and all the demons surrounding it. Yes, it involves that word 'acceptance' again.

As Navalny wrote in his prison diary when his wife Yulia visited:

I do not want to sound dramatic, but I think there's a high probability I'll never get out of here. Even if everything starts falling apart, they will bump me off at the first side the regime is collapsing. They will poison me'. 'I know', she said with a nod, in a voice that was calm and firm, 'I was thinking of that myself'. At that moment I wanted to seize her in my arms and hug her joyfully, as hard as I could. That was so great! No tears! It was one of those moments when you realise you have found the right person. 'Or she found you'. 'Let's just decide for ourselves that this is most likely what's going to happen. Let's accept it as a base scenario and arrange our lives on that basis.

'If things turn out better, that will be marvellous, but we won't count on it or have ill founded hopes'.

(extract from *The New Yorker*, October 11, 2024)

This is what I would call complete acceptance, and although Alexei Navalny was exceptional, I think we all have the germ of acceptance like this inside.

The adaptation to internal negative affect is one of the most difficult parts of personal adjustment. Many of those with persistent anxiety and other mood disturbance regard it as an affective (affect is the same as emotion) illness, a mood disorder that has to be treated directly, and often aggressively, with both psychological and drug treatments. But, as I have argued elsewhere (Tyrer, 2018; Tyrer & Baldwin, 2006), it is wrong to casually satisfy the need for a diagnostic label by summarising this as generalised anxiety disorder or dysthymia and think you have the condition clean and dusted. If you have continual anxiety and nervous symptoms from childhood onward, if these are linked to lack of self-confidence, avoidance of situations perceived as stressful, and a long-standing tendency to rely on others for support, you are not suffering from an anxiety disorder; you have a primary personality problem in which negative affectivity is the dominant domain. In the past, we gave this range of conditions the general term of neurosis. This was an umbrella term covering a wide range, but a large proportion can be viewed as having the general neurotic syndrome (see Chapter 16), a chronic disorder that is treated unsuccessfully by a panoply of treatments, largely drugs called selective serotonin reuptake inhibitors (SSRIs) in current practice and which tends to get worse, not better, as you age (Tyrer et al., 2022).

We should not give up trying to find better ways of treating this condition, made insufferable when depression is present in equal degree, but we should not abandon the idea of adaptation. 'I've had this condition all my life', many of my patients tell me. 'If there was a way of adapting, I would have found it by now'. But our bodies do not like persistent disturbance, and if we ourselves do not find a way of compensating for it, they will take the responsibility to adapt in maladaptive forms.

One of these is to take refuge in alcohol or drugs. This is one of the easiest ways to remove the whole range of unpleasant emotions. Alcohol is a major depressant of the nervous system, so much so that it can cut off life support systems altogether in excessive dosage, but it appears to lift depressed mood in smaller quantities, a lovely feeling that does not last. I am not dwelling on the risks of substance use here except to add that their 'positive affectivity' components should be treasured in small doses only.

Table 9.1 Adaptation guide to negative affectivity

Form of adaptation	Nature of adaptation
Goals	Decide which of the priorities you have is the most important and stick to it. Try and achieve an internal locus of control.
Relationships	Keep most contact with those you love and respect and do not rush into others.
Lifestyle	Reassess your life; decide who you want to be and follow the selected path.
Occupation	Stick to the areas in which you excel; do not be diverted.
Leisure pursuits	With your personality, you need to avoid feelings of humiliation, so generally avoid competitive events unless you are very skilled, and go for ones that are calming and stabilise your mood.
Conflict avoidance	The people who annoy you should be avoided unless they are ones you love, in which case they and you must be trained to avoid the subjects that give rise to conflict

Guidance for adaptation to negative affectivity

Goals

Goals are important in life, even though at times they do not seem to have much relevance. When Captain Tom Moore decided to raise money for the NHS by walking the length of his garden 100 times before his 100th birthday, he hoped to raise £1000; in the end, he raised £17 million. Some goal, some success. But, no matter what the object, having a goal, or more than one without being too greedy, is good for your health and self-esteem. Even if the goal is a tiny one—to travel on your own to a garden centre to buy that pot plant that would look fantastic in the front window—it is still an important milestone. In those smothered by the dead hand of negative affectivity, goals on which to focus attention are even more important.

Relationships

The relationships of those with strong negative affectivity tend to be limited but can become too restricted. Adapting to them can include expanding their scope in a way that still retains an internal locus of control. So if you are a card player and like whist or bridge, the possibility of expanding your group to four could be a low-stress option, bringing others into your orbit with all having clear roles.

Lifestyle and occupation

The concept behind nidotherapy is the nest: the soft, comfortable, and familiar environment in which we can curl up and feel safe from the world outside. That is particularly attractive to the nervous and insecure, and it often serves them well. But when it fails, a new venture is needed, and adaptation may be difficult. When this becomes necessary, the familiar supportive elements need to be retained as much as possible. A good home has to accommodate all your habits and your whims. The same is true of your occupation, but only a few can make it quite as snug as the home.

Conflict avoidance

Open conflict is very troubling to negative affectivity. It can lead to rumination, self-doubt, depression, and despair. No matter what the cause or the justification, these consequences will tend to follow. So such people need to be protected from the pain of these occasions, and this is where those whom the person is dependent on and close to have to deflect and intervene to ward off the consequences.

References

Boswell J (1791). *The Life of Dr Johnson*. Abridged as *Everybody's Boswell*, edited by Frank Morley. London: G Bell & Son, 1930.

Eliot TS (1915). *The Love Song of J. Alfred Prufrock*. Chicago: Poetry.

Hovenkamp-Hermelink JHM, Jeronimus BF, van der Veen DC, Spinhoven P, Penninx BWJH, Schoevers RA, et al. (2019). Differential associations of locus of control with anxiety, depression and life-events: a five-wave, nine-year study to test stability and change. *Journal of Affective Disorders*, 253, 26–34.

Rotter JB (1990). Internal versus external control of reinforcement. A case history of a variable. *American Psychologist*, 45, 489–493.

Tyrer P (2009). *Nidotherapy: Harmonising the Environment with the Patient*. London: RCPsych Press.

Tyrer P (2018). Against the Stream: Generalised anxiety disorder (GAD): a redundant diagnosis. *BJPsych Bulletin*, 42, 69–71.

Tyrer P & Baldwin D (2006). Generalised anxiety disorder. *Lancet*, 368, 2156–2166.

Tyrer P, Ferguson B, Fowler-Dixon R, & Kelemen A (1990). A plea for the diagnosis of hypochondriacal personality disorder. *Journal of Psychosomatic Research*, 34, 637–642.

Tyrer P, Seivewright N, & Seivewright H (1999). Long term outcome of hypochondriacal personality disorder. *Journal of Psychosomatic Research*, 46, 177–185.

Tyrer P, Tyrer H, Johnson T, & Yang M (2022). Thirty year outcome of anxiety and depressive disorders and personality status: comprehensive evaluation of mixed symptoms and the general neurotic syndrome in the follow-up of a randomised controlled trial. *Psychological Medicine*, 52, 3999–4008.

Chapter 10

Adapting to the detachment domain

There are many who have a strong detached domain in their personalities who are well adjusted and adapted and so do not need any further help. They are self-sufficient, independent people who have clear direction in life and do not rely on other people as they are confident in their own abilities. The older adjective for detached personalities was 'schizoid', a somewhat cruel word that can be crudely translated as a staging post on the way to schizophrenia, but it is easy to see how wrong such a label can be. More recently, detachment has become linked to autism, now reformulated as autism spectrum disorder.

Steve Silberman (2015) has beautifully reformulated this large group into a cracking new construction, 'neurotribes', or 'a convivial population of loners'. Far from being isolated from society, these people have now become innovators and developers. They are often celebrated. In Silberman's words:

> [T]heir equivalents in the mid-twentieth century aimed telescopes at the stars, built radios from mail-order kits, or blew up beakers in the garage. In the past forty years, some members of this tribe have migrated from the margins of society to the mainstream and currently work at companies like Facebook, Apple, and Google. Along the way, they have refashioned pop culture in their own image; now it's cool to be obsessed with dinosaurs, periodic tables and Doctor Who—at any age.
>
> (Silberman, p. 3)

I personally do not feel we have quite got this subject properly described in either popular or specialist literature. We have, in my view correctly, rid ourselves of the diagnosis of Asperger's syndrome, a condition nicely resurrected by Lorna Wing in 1981 but now absorbed into autistic spectrum disorder, but we are still thinking of autism as a disease. Even bowdlerising the description as 'neurodiversity', which only means we all have different nervous systems, gives an impression of pathology that should not really

DOI: 10.4324/9781003560630-10

be there. The idea behind the language of autistic spectrum disorder is a good one—it extends across the full range of 100% autistic to no autistic features at all—but when we euphemistically venture that a patient is 'somewhere on the autistic spectrum', we are not saying they are near the 0% but see them as a considerable distance away.

Lorna Wing wrote that there is no doubt 'Asperger syndrome can be regarded as a form of schizoid personality', but she questioned whether such a label was of any value. I agree, as you will guess without too much difficulty after what I have written elsewhere in this book, but when it comes to the general notion of personality, I differ. If we are going to take the ICD-11 classification of personality disturbance seriously, we can avoid a lot of unnecessary labelling. Diagnosis necessarily compartmentalises people, giving them all a collective ownership that is only partly correct and sometimes plain wrong. We can do the same with the diagnosis of personality disturbance but do not need to except at the extreme end of the range when legal and forensic requirements force us to make categorical judgments that determine a person's fate. For others, we can put most people on a spectrum of individual oddity that makes them all different but also more interesting.

The detached group of personalities are quite in place on this spectrum, dotted across the range. But some have difficulties that tend to be accentuated if they are not resolved. For those who have a measure of personality difficulty, troubles knock more loudly. A major disturbance in life, rejection by a lover, failure in a job application, an insulting dismissal, even abuse on social media can have a devastating impact. At this time, for many people, a period of detachment and reflection is not something to despise. As the perceptive psychoanalyst Anthony Storr puts it, '[I]n a culture in which interpersonal relationships are generally considered to provide the answer to every form of distress, it is sometimes difficult to persuade well-meaning helpers that solitude can be as therapeutic as emotional support' (Storr, 1988).

If we recall the famous words of John Donne, 'no man is an island', there are some with strong detachment tendencies who become unmoored so far away from others in the ocean of humanity they suffer the consequence of the isolation that follows. Prolonged isolation leads to loss of social skills and inability to relate, and this leads others to avoid contact and magnify the isolation. Independence of mind then becomes pigheadedness and stupidity and leads to further rejection from society. The person often responds by rejecting other people angrily, and this rapidly moves toward paranoia.

Once paranoia has set into relationships with others it feeds on itself voraciously, adding more and more to the many people who are rejected as personal adversaries, people wrongly perceived as having personal grudges and aggressive motives. It is in these situations that violence may be shown. In prisons there is a belief that those with detached personalities and autism have a greater propensity to violence, but it is not well founded and those that are violent usually have other pathologies that are more likely to be linked.

(Långström et al., 2009)

But the impression given to the outside world is not a friendly one. The detached person's home is often the last bastion of defence against a hostile world and can become a fortress, a shield against society. One just needs to read about the number of disputes, some ending in death, that are connected to the physical boundaries that set us apart from our neighbours. Fast-growing trees such as leylandii have a lot to answer for in stories of human conflict.

Even detached personalities need to have contact with others to prevent their views and behaviour from being untethered from reality. To some extent, this can be offset by having regular contact with news and other media that inform without the need to engage, but for those who are completely alone, this is never enough.

Mental health professionals will never have patients with detached personalities queuing to see them because they no longer wish to be mistrustful and paranoid and want to have therapy to correct these feelings. No, it is more than likely that they will include health professionals as players in the paranoid orchestra who have deliberately played the wrong notes to upset them. So how do we advise and adapt?

The first requirement is to have what John Bowlby called an 'attachment figure'. He developed his theories of attachment in his studies of very young children, and the main attachment figure in his theory is, most naturally, a mother (Bowlby, 1969). But it does not have to be, and when Bowlby reflected on his own upbringing in an upper-middle-class family in the early 1900s, he realised his main attachment figure was his nanny, Minnie, who left the household when John was four and left him devastated.

A detached personality needs to have some form of external attachment to maintain a sense of societal balance. Human face-to-face attachments are always preferable, but sometimes digital online options can be substituted, and in the future, artificial intelligence (AI) may provide the kind of contact that is consensual with the personality and yet connected more closely to the wider world.

In giving advice here, I have to admit that it may have the same impact as talking in a large empty hall; you stretch to hear a response, but the voice you hear is just your own echo. Detached personalities do not queue to listen; it's thumbs down for advice they do not want. But they can still

Table 10.1 Adaptation guide to detachment

Form of adaptation	Nature of adaptation
Goals	Detached personalities are usually good at setting goals, so long as they are feasible.
Relationships	Limit these as much as you wish but still keep an attachment figure with you.
Lifestyle	Aim for healthy independence and a good life balance.
Occupation	Find tasks where you can be unrestricted, and your wish to work alone and largely unsupervised is respected.
Leisure pursuits	Choose activities you can perform alone or ones with few people and clear rules (e.g., chess).
Conflict avoidance	Plan ahead to avoid situations when conflict can arise.

adapt, and others they know can help greatly too. They can read this section, and they can listen to the small number of people they can trust—and then start to make a few tentative changes.

Goals

Many who are independent have clear goals that are followed with stubborn determination. Sometimes this degree of independence is highly successful. Thomas Jackson was a confederate general in the American Civil War. We have mixed opinions about those who fought on the confederate side as they were warring to retain slavery, but nobody would deny that there was bravery on both sides. Thomas did not listen to the advice of experts. He made his own decisions, including help in getting what would now be called a topographical analysis of the battlefield (i.e., an accurate record of every hill, valley, gully, and stream) so he knew where to deploy his troops. He was able to hide them and unleash them at the right time to surprise the enemy. He had a detached personality and, though highly intelligent, was very eccentric; when lecturing to students, he held one arm high in the air to encourage its growth. But his determination and analytical view of warfare turned out to be very successful.

Relationships

Many people who are detached find relationships intolerable because they are so unpredictable. I was once asked to advise over the best management for a highly successful professor who had suddenly fallen in performance. He had carried out very original ground-breaking work in his laboratory work with rats. As often happens in universities, he was promoted to become head of a much bigger department. In this role, he had to advise and supervise research colleagues but also help staff from other sections and act as a mentor and guide to many students.

But he was not equipped for this role. His personal behaviour upset many, he could be rude and short tempered, and many complaints were made. He became even more crotchety and difficult, so a review of his performance was arranged. When I saw him, it was clear that he agreed he was unhappy in his work. He told me he found it very difficult to understand many of the problems raised by the students as, in his words, 'they were not problems that would ever occur to me'.

The answer to the difficulty was quite simple. Rat behaviour was much more predictable than human behaviour, so he should return to the laboratory.

Lifestyle

People who are detached need to organise their lives as there are few who could do it for them. But this fits their need to be in control of their lives. Most successful detached personalities have a strong internal locus of control; they have the levers to determine all aspects of their lives as they have chosen which levers to use and their importance right from the start. Sometimes they may go awry, but others should not be needed to bring them back into line.

Occupation

As Steve Silberman reminded us, those with detached personalities in this digital age are not on the edge of society; they are its prime movers. Steve Jobs, the founder of Apple and Mac computers, was an outsider who dropped out of school and college and pursued a lopsided education involving literature, Buddhism, calligraphy, and electronics at different times without any formal guidance. This did not matter; he was outside the frame of convention, and standard instruction passed him by without looking. His independent detached personality won the day and made a great deal of money for his company.

Not many detached personalities can be like Steve Jobs, but we must give all of them the chance to flourish.

Conflict avoidance

Many people with detached personalities come into conflict with others because their views are very different from conventionally accepted ones. So it is difficult to avoid conflict in such circumstances. The best advice is to anticipate conflict by going in a different direction so it never arises.

References

Bowlby J (1969). *Attachment and Loss, Volume 1: Attachment*. New York: Basic Books.

Långström N, Grann M, Ruchkin V, Sjöstedt G, & Fazel S (2009). Risk factors for violent offending in autism spectrum disorder: a national study of hospitalized individuals. *Journal of Interpersonal Violence*, 24, 1358–1370.

Silberman S (2015). *Neurotribes. The Legacy of Autism and the Future of Neurodiversity*. Random House.

Storr A (1988). *Solitude: A Return to the Self*. The Free Press.

Wing L (1981). Asperger's syndrome: a clinical account. *Psychological Medicine*, 11, 115–129.

Chapter 11

Adapting to the dissociality domain

The dissociality domain represents a more difficult one to promote adaptation as those who have this characteristic most prominently are not always keen on losing it. Put another way, they are very much in favour of adaptation for their own needs but usually at odds with the needs of others. The essence of antisociality is in the name; it is in conflict with society. It does not follow the same rules and takes great pleasure from breaking them. In this context, adaptation then becomes an exercise in more successful rule-breaking. In the words of a recent comprehensive text:

> A key characteristic of antisocial individuals, particularly those with high levels of psychopathic traits, namely, is that they lack the motivation to engage in an empathic way with others. It is not surprising that these individuals sometimes report that they feel fundamentally disconnected from their social environment. This does not mean that their behaviour is unmotivated or that they fail to engage with other people; on the contrary, it means only that their motives, particularly when engaging with others, are different from those of most people, and are viewed by most as deviant.
>
> (Howard & Duggan, 2022, p. 37)

The three main features of the dissocial domain can be summarised as the three I's: insensitivity, infringement, and injury, a somewhat shorter list than Robert Hare's psychopathy checklist (PCL-R) (Table 11.1).

These encompass the central features of antisociality and psychopathy. Because we are all still puzzled about the best ways of treating people with these features, there are repeated attempts to understand the motivation and thinking behind these patterns of behaviour. These have some value, but I suspect they are more interesting to crime writers than therapists as they appear to promote explanation more than intervention.

I now have to introduce the dark tetrad of personality traits, a term that sounds as though it may have come from *Star Wars*—'It is no good, Obi Wen Kenobi, the dark tetrad are by my side; you cannot win against their

DOI: 10.4324/9781003560630-11

Table 11.1 The three *I*'s of dissociality (after Tyrer et al., 2021)

Characteristic	
Insensitivity	The ability of some to disregard the humanity of others; to commit execrable acts against a person without any remorse
Infringement	The violation of basic rights of others
Injury	Injury and unjustified physical and mental aggression, used as a means of control

wily machinations'. They comprise psychopathy, narcissism, Machiavellianism, and sadism. The first three began life as the dark triad (Paulhus & Williams, 2002); sadism was added later to make up the tetrad (Paulhus, 2014). These terms have been embraced by those who look for antisociality in commerce, in business, and in large organisations rather than in medical clinics. Those who have the dark tetrad are typically described as callous, cynical, dishonest, manipulative, self-aggrandising, and self-absorbed and always act in favour of self-interest and at the expense of others.

Working toward positive adaptation to society is not an easy task in this scenario. The advantages of selfishness are immediate; those of altruism are delayed. Most of the claimed treatments for antisocial behaviour are not carried out in clinics with people queueing at the entrances; they are given to incarcerated people who have time on their hands and feel by taking part in treatment programmes they may get an earlier release.

But there is one exception. A modification of mentalisation-based treatment (MBT) that focuses on the mental and relational processes in the personality rather than violent and other aggressive behaviours has shown encouraging signs (Bateman et al., 2016; Bateman, 2022), and a full trial is being published. It may be a harbinger of things to come.

The NICE guidelines for the management of antisocial personality disorder (National Institute for Health and Care Excellence, 2009) did not express any view about successful treatments and could only give general advice (Box 11.1):

Box 11.1. General advice about management of antisocial personality disorder (National Institute for Health and Care Excellence, 2009, revised 2013)

1.1.3 Autonomy and choice
1.1.3.1 Work in partnership with people with antisocial personality disorder to develop their autonomy and promote choice by:
- ensuring that they remain actively involved in finding solutions to their problems, including during crises
- encouraging them to consider the different treatment options and life choices available to them, and the consequences of the choices they make.

We currently have to rely on work carried out in institutions where the motivation of those taking part is far from clear. This population is not likely to be a representative one, but as we have more data in prison populations, including adaptation strategies, this is worth examining in detail first.

It is not easy to convert antisocial to prosocial when so much of the fuel of dissociality is aggression. Anger against a person, a group, or a system is a powerful force. In nidotherapy, we have not made much progress with prisoners, partly because the rules of prisons do not allow the testing out of new environments if they are perceived as having any risk attached (Spencer et al., 2010), coupled with a general suspiciousness of new ideas in the one prison (NM Wormwood Scrubs) where we proposed our intervention.

One approach that shows some similarities to nidotherapy, even though it has mainly been used with sex offenders, is the good lives model (Ward, 2002). This acknowledges the importance of the focus on criminality but avoids the attention normally given to risk by attempting to foster the development of positive goals that are wanted and can be achieved without the need for antisocial actions. The good lives model (GLM) argues that all meaningful human actions represent attempts to secure goals, which may be the acquisition of goods, reward in other activities such as sports, the completion of valued tasks, or life satisfaction. The GLM argues that people who are antisocial follow these goals in harmful ways because of their past experiences and recent behaviour. The approach of the GLM is to reinforce social and psychological resources in a way that moves them in a prosocial direction. Once this has become established, further development continues when achievements follow that are intrinsically beneficial and reinforcing.

It could be argued that GLM and nidotherapy are similar in this respect and could create a model of adaptation for dissociality. Both are based on active collaboration between therapist and patient, with emphasis on a strong therapeutic alliance. GLM explicitly emphasises individualised treatment, including development of a good lives plan that is designed and developed collaboratively with the offender, although with sex offenders, this may be carried out in groups (Willis et al., 2014). Both nidotherapy and GLM place emphasis on the individual in deciding on change, so personal agency is encouraged, with the therapist acting only as a facilitator, not as a decision-maker. Both approaches use the person's strengths in helping choose changes that can are feasible and possible within the repertoire of the person's abilities. Finally, both approaches take account of environmental resources and opportunities in reducing offending (in the case of GLM) or improving patients' mental health (in the case of nidotherapy).

This sounds to be a good way forward. The difficulty I have with adopting comes down to motivation. In our work, we were involved in evaluating the Dangerous and Severe Personality Disorder programme set up in the UK in 2000 as a bold attempt both to detect those who were most dangerous to society and to provide effective treatments. The Home Office, Department of Health, NHS, and Prison Service all supported it, but not the Royal College of Psychiatrists or the Mental Health Alliance, representing nearly 100 voluntary bodies, who felt there was a real danger that people could be wrongly incarcerated in the programme without reason. We found this to be justified (Tyrer et al., 2009).

By 2010, the programme had cost £480M but is still continuing in a less expensive form, particularly in the prisons, where it received a much warmer reception than in the special hospitals where it was introduced:

> [P]articipants within the prison system, although critical of aspects of the regime, seemed more willing to accept that as a prisoner there was a reason why they were incarcerated, other than simply as a waiting area for therapy. All the participants met the criteria for DSPD (severe personality disorder, directly linked to a high risk of further serious offending), yet those managed within the hospital system were more focused on their entitlement to treatment than their role as offender.
>
> (Sinclair et al., 2012, p. 253)

This reflects the different expectations of patients and prisoners, even though at first sight they appear to be the same.

In all the centres, both prisons and special hospitals, there were psychological treatment programmes not very different from the good lives model (which was incorporated later), but it was very difficult to determine if they were effective. As our research evaluation was independent of the main functioning of the programme, the prisoners and patients could afford to be honest when talking to us about the value of these interventions. Unfortunately, there was a healthy degree of cynicism about many of the programmes. Comments such as 'It's obvious what they are trying to do, and I'll go along with it if its going to lead to my early release' and 'I am very happy in this prison and do not particularly want to leave, so I am going to volunteer for as many of the treatment programmes as I can so I can stay longer' were not entirely moving in the prosocial direction.

The value of the Good Lives Model can only really be assessed through careful research enquiries about its long-term outcome compared with other programmes. These will be difficult to set up and follow through, but until we have good data, we will remain whistling in the dark, clutching at straws of efficacy without ever being certain they are real. In our considered summary of the programme after ten years, we concluded,

> [The costs of the enterprise are very high and it is likely that decision-makers in the future will consider the level of gain to be

unjustified in terms of cost. Clearly there are some gains, and much has been learnt since the programme began, but if the experiment is to continue in any form the additional expenditure has to be linked to results, and these are conspicuously lacking to date.

A randomised controlled trial has recently been published whose results can be interpreted both as highly heartening and mildly depressing. This study, set in prisons, assessed nearly 2000 male convicted prisoners and recruited 313 of them to the trial, randomly allocating half of them to an intensive course of mentalisation-based therapy (MBT) and the other half to the standard follow-up input of probation. Those allocated to MBT were offered 12 months of weekly 75 minute MBT groups and monthly individual sessions of 50 minutes each. Follow-up assessments were carried out at 3 month intervals up to 24 months and final follow-up, in which assessments were complicated by the COVID pandemic, was carried out at 24–36 months. Those allocated to MBT had more offences initially than the probation group but this was probably because they were released from prison earlier (reasons for this not quite clear) but overall there was a significantly greater reduction in aggression and in offences in the MBT group, most of which was lost at follow-up. Less than a third of the initial probation group completed follow-up assessments and less than half completed them in the MBT group.

(Fonagy et al., 2025)

Despite all these difficulties, the trial was certainly a success carried out under very difficult circumstances in a population that all knew in advance would challenge good follow-up rates. An additional strong positive from the trial was evidence that the intervention was cost effective, but this might have been largely related to the earlier release of prisoners in the MBT group with associated cost savings.

But why is it necessary to add the comment that the results are mildly depressing? It is the longer-term outcome that is troubling. Despite very heavy intensive therapy, gains were not maintained over time, and a large proportion of both groups did not engage with either arm of the trial or complete assessments. It could be argued that the results are not surprising, as it is suspected that those with the greatest need for intervention do not engage (McMurran et al., 2010; Mathlin et al., 2021), and other trials in antisocial populations have shown that benefits are quickly lost (Howard & Duggan, 2022; Mohajerin & Howard, 2024).

Gains have been made, but how should we judge these results overall? I can best interpret them in the form of a story.

There are two adjacent countries, Sparse and Plenty. Those who live in Sparse are in a desert landscape; very little can be grown in the way of crops, and the population is always at the brink of starvation. By contrast, the citizens of Plenty live in a verdant landscape of fields and rivers and enjoy excellent food and a high standard of living. The government of Plenty looked across at Sparse and felt sorry for their plight. They decided, with the agreement of the government of Sparse, to help by sending a delegation of cooks with food from Plenty to teach the principles of good cooking and husbandry to the Sparse people. By the end of six months, everybody in Sparse was happy as, for the first time, they were well fed and knew how to prepare and cook good food.

The delegation from Plenty returned home and were praised for their generosity and cooking exploits. A year later, the delegation from Plenty visited again as they wished to write a report on the progress that had been made. Sadly, everything had returned to the previous state of semi-starvation. Ill-fed children were scouring the streets for food, men were digging unsuccessfully for wells, and mothers were grinding husks of corn over and over again to obtain a few grains of flour. The cooking gains had all been lost as no effort had been made to improve the harsh environment of Sparse.

To extend this allegory, if the principles of nidotherapy had also been applied to Sparse at the same time as their cookery training, the outcome could have been very different. If drip irrigation, efficient rainwater harvesting, and the planting of trees and drought resistant-crops had all been introduced with the cooking course, the new produce that was harvested could have maintained and reinforced the cookery gains. Not only the cooking needed to change; the environment needed adjustment also.

Concentrating the resources on those who are clearly motivated and determined to overcome their propensity to re-offend may be one way forward, but it is clear that this would only include a minority of those currently in the 'programme' (Tyrer et al., 2010). Improving the environment can be applied to all.

Richard Howard (personal comment) sees merit in combining nidotherapy with a GLM-based intervention in the antisocial population. The latter can be initiated while the offender/patient is detained, either in prison or forensic psychiatry, and would be aimed at developing a new 'good life' plan to be followed after their release. Nidotherapy could be applied following release into the community, aimed at improving the offender's mental health. In combination, both should foster the patient/offender's desistance from crime and improve their mental health.

Because I am not yet convinced about the way forward for this domain, I am not providing an adaptation guide.

References

Bateman A, O'Connell J, Lorenzini N, Gardner T, & Fonagy P (2016). A randomised controlled trial of mentalization-based treatment versus structured clinical management for patients with comorbid borderline personality disorder and antisocial personality disorder. *BMC Psychiatry*, 16, 304.

Bateman AW (2022). Mentalizing and group psychotherapy: a novel treatment for antisocial personality disorder. *American Journal of Psychotherapy*, 75, 32–37.

Fonagy P, Simes E, Yirmiya K, Wason J, Barrett B, Frater A, et al. (2025). Mentalisation-based treatment for antisocial personality disorder in males convicted of an offence on community probation in England and Wales (Mentalization for Offending Adult Males, MOAM): a multicentre, assessor-blinded, randomised controlled trial. *Lancet Psychiatry*, 12, 208–219.

Howard R & Duggan C (2022). *Antisocial Personality: Theory, Research, Treatment*. Cambridge University Press.

Mathlin G, Freestone M, Taylor C, & Shaw J (2021). Offenders with personality disorder who fail to progress: a case-control study using partial least squares structural equation modeling path analysis. *JMIRx Med*, 2, e27907.

McMurran M, Huband N, & Overton E (2010). Non-completion of personality disorder treatments: a systematic review of correlates, consequences, and interventions. *Clinical Psychology Review*, 30(3), 277–287.

Mohajerin B & Howard RC (2024). Effects of two treatments on interpersonal, affective, and lifestyle features of psychopathy and emotion dysregulation. *Personality and Mental Health*, 18, 43–59.

Paulhus DL (2014). Toward a taxonomy of dark personalities. *Current Directions in Psychological Science*, 23, 421–426.

Paulhus DL & Williams KM (2002). The Dark Triad of personality: narcissism, Machiavellianism and psychopathy. *Journal of Research in Personality*, 36, 556–563.

Sinclair J, Willmott L, Fitzpatrick R, Burns T, & Yiend J; IDEA Group (2012). Patients' experience of dangerous and severe personality disorder services: qualitative interview study. *British Journal of Psychiatry*, 200, 252–253.

Spencer S-J, Rutter D, & Tyrer P (2010). Integration of nidotherapy into the management of mental illness and antisocial personality: a qualitative study. *International Journal of Social Psychiatry*, 56, 50–59.

Tyrer P, Cooper S, Rutter D, Seivewright H, Duggan C, Maden T, et al. (2009). The assessment of dangerous and severe personality disorder: lessons from a randomised controlled trial linked to qualitative analysis. *Journal of Forensic Psychiatry & Psychology*, 20, 132–146.

Tyrer P, Duggan C, Cooper S, Crawford M, Seivewright H, Rutter D, et al. (2010). The successes & failures of the DSPD experiment: the assessment & management of severe personality disorder. *Medicine, Science & the Law*, 50, 95–99.

Tyrer P, Farnam A, Zahmatkesh A, & Sanatinia R (2021). Conceptual and definitional issues. In: DW Black & N Kolla (eds.), *Textbook of Antisocial Personality Disorder*. Washington, DC: American Psychiatric Press.

Ward T (2002). Good lives and the rehabilitation of offenders: promises and problems. *Aggression and Violent Behavior*, 7, 513–528.

Willis GM, Ward T, & Levenson JS (2014). The good lives model (GLM): an evaluation of GLM operationalization in North American treatment programs. *Sex Abuse*, 26, 58–81.

Chapter 12

Adapting to the disinhibited domain

This is a rather more difficult task than adapting to the other domains. Impulsiveness is a trait, but it is an episodic one, and it is often bound up with negative affectivity (emotional impulsiveness) and dissociality (the impulsiveness of gain). It is also a core feature of attention deficit-hyperactivity disorder (ADHD), and the attraction of ADHD as an alternative diagnosis to personality disorder may be one of the reasons the diagnosis of ADHD is increasing in prevalence (now more than 10% in children in the US) (Li et al., 2023).

Emotional impulsiveness

In Chapter 4, I separated emotional dysregulation from the other domains of personality and suggested it should be regarded as a mental disorder, not as a domain trait. Emotional impulsiveness is part of emotional dysregulation and so has to be dealt with similarly. Emotional impulsivity has never had evolutionary benefits or created any kind of gain; it is one of the reasons so many people see it as a negative aspect of the borderline concept, and reaction to it is often a strong promoter of stigma.

The impulsiveness of gain

The impulsiveness associated with immediate gain is a personality characteristic. The apparent gain may be financial—stealing, cheating, robbing, fraud—but may also be associated with more subtle purposes, changing the tenor of a relationship by an impulsive kiss, interrupting a meeting with an angry interjection in order to get attention, showing off in a game of cards by staking too high, driving too fast to get to a destination before a rival.

If you can recognise these tendencies in advance and can have an internal message 'think again' ready for transmission at all times, this may help. Having a rubber band around your wrist that, at impulsive times, you can

DOI: 10.4324/9781003560630-12

Table 12.1 Adaptation guide to impulsiveness

Form of adaptation	Nature of adaptation
Goals	Do not decide on the goals you want to achieve in a hurry. Give them great thought and ask advice from others if you can.
Relationships	Do not make major decisions in your relationships without considering all the consequences that may follow.
Lifestyle	Limit drug and alcohol consumption to the minimum; do not take any without thought.
Occupation	Look for certainty in your work; do not be seduced by novelty.
Leisure pursuits	Avoid activities that pose extra risk to body, soul, and bank balance.
Conflict avoidance	Anticipate conflict situations by avoidance wherever possible; when inevitable, rehearse as much as possible in advance.

pull, let go, and sting can be another method of reminding you that dangerous territory lies ahead.

Goals

Solid goals are golden goals; they take time and thought to develop. Impulsiveness and disinhibition tend to sabotage them and introduce short-term gains that are counter-productive. It is important not to be swayed by them. Think again, think again.

Relationships

Impulsiveness is a powerful creator and destroyer of relationships; it may only take an instant. Often it becomes very difficult to retract. In the past, there were many complex court cases involving breach of promise—in most cases, they were won by the female partner—Eva Haraldsted of Denmark being the last example in 1969. She successfully sued George Best, a well-established impulsivist. Nowadays it is easier to wriggle out of responsibility in these matters, but we still need to be reminded of the impact of impulsive decisions that have long-term consequences.

Lifestyle and occupation

It is difficult to give advice about working patterns to people who have a natural tendency to look for variety and novelty around every corner. But there are professions such as acting and many jobs in the media which are littered with variety and change and so are attractive to those of impulsive bent. This can work well provided there are other elements that are much more grounded and stable in life.

Leisure pursuits and conflict avoidance

A typical person with a strong impulsive trait will tend to pursue leisure activities that are to some extent risky and likely to provoke conflict. There is absolutely nothing wrong with this, and this impulsiveness is shown in sport and other games; it is probably safer than expressing it in other settings. A major hazard is the possible increase in the consumption of alcohol and drugs as part of these leisure activities, and many of them should carry a health warning to those who are impulsive.

Reference

Li Y, Yan X, Li Q, Li Q, Xu G, Lu J, & Yang W (2023). Prevalence and trends in diagnosed ADHD among US children and adolescents, 2017–2022. *JAMA Network Open*, 6, e2336872.

Chapter 13

Adapting to the anankastic domain

The anankastic domain is the only one of the five domains of personality that most people treasure. Being hard working, diligent, and productive appeals to everybody, but only at a level of moderation that does not impair performance and can harmonise with others. For many people, the ability to have a little more anankastia would be seen as an advantage, but this does not mean it is free from problems.

The business magnate, film-maker, and aircraft designer Howard Hughes spent a large amount of his fortune in creating what he considered (wrongly) to be a completely germ-free environment as he was so concerned about the dangers of infection. His staff were trained in ludicrous methods to promote his wishes. So, for example, when he received canned food, his staff were first asked to put the can in running warm water, then remove the label with a brush and special soap bars. Afterward, the can was soaked to remove all germs, and the bottom of the can treated in the same way as the rest before it could be passed on to him. Because he was at the top of a pyramid of complete control, he was able to maintain this behaviour for years, usually by living in and moving from hotel to hotel until he died.

No amount of advice could change his views, although at a preconscious level, he probably recognised his behaviour was not grounded in environmental reality, and the Howard Hughes Medical Institute that he founded shows that part of him was fully grounded; this is now one of the largest medical research bodies in the world.

A nidotherapist would have made little progress with Howard. He was very keen on innovation but not if it was directed at him. If he had been exposed to any suggestions to improve his health, he would probably have responded by setting up a research organisation to treat every other sufferer apart from himself.

In most biographies, Howard Hughes is described as suffering from obsessive-compulsive disorder (OCD). This is incorrect. Those with OCD want to be rid of their obsessions; Howard only promoted them

DOI: 10.4324/9781003560630-13

to absurdity. He had strong elements of anankastia in his personality and the very strong personality strength of independence, and this combination of personality characteristics made him both brilliant and ridiculous.

We must not run down the advantages of the anankastic trait. It helps in life, and people who have it as a prominent characteristic live longer than all others (Graham et al., 2017). Yet the other side of anankastia is stubbornness, rigidity, obstinacy, persnicketiness, excessive attention to rules, and the inability to alter behaviour in the light of circumstances. These features can become a subject of ridicule. There is a side-splitting joke told by Bob Newhart, the celebrated American comedian, about an obsessional new guard, Jake, at the Empire State Building in New York. Jake has been very diligent in following his training for the post and wants to do everything right. But he is faced with an unexpected event that throws him off balance. A large ape by the name of King Kong (he does not know the name yet, but he will shortly) is beginning to climb up the building.

Jake phones his supervisor.

'I hate to bother you at home, sir, but something has come up that is not in my guard's manual. There's an ape's toe sticking through the window'.

He is given various pieces of advice after following the rule book carefully. He is advised to dislodge King Kong's toe but fails, and he is then advised to go and strike King Kong in the face. This sounds reasonable, but Jake has a problem that only the obsessional will recognise.

'I'd like to do that sir, but his face is on the 19th floor, and that's too far up. My jurisdiction only extends to his navel'.

The major problems arising from obsessionality are three: the need to control, the need to be perfect, and the need to compete and win. These can all be adapted positively, and as those who are anankastic are persistent, adaptation should succeed.

Table 13.1 Adaptation guide to anankastia

Form of adaptation	Nature of adaptation
Goals	Set goals that are attainable; do not be too ambitious.
Relationships	Do not be swayed too much by your own personal traits; it may serve you better to have close relationships with those of opposite tendencies.
Lifestyle	Try and preserve a good work-life balance; do not let it become lopsided.
Occupation	Go for the best, but do not let it take over your life.
Leisure pursuits	Try and be as active as possible in your leisure time.
Conflict avoidance	Learn how to defuse.

Goals

Obsessional people are good at setting goals, providing they are attainable. Problems can arise when there is a block in progress. There is a tendency then for more and more effort being expended on overcoming the barrier instead of finding a different way around it. Isaac Newton, the brilliant mathematician and experimenter who discovered the secrets of light and gravity and invented calculus, spent many of the latter years of his life attempting to turn base metals into gold. Because he had been so successful previously, he was convinced he could find the philosopher's stone that would transmute metals. But he was ignorant of the molecular structure of atoms, and all his efforts failed, but he never stopped trying.

Relationships

It is the natural state of the anankast to be fully in control in all parts of life, but when it comes to relationships, this can run into difficulties. It is all very well having full control of your own life but quite another having full control of the lives of others. This can be perfectly appropriate in the care of very young children and of elderly people with dementia, but not for those who have the ability to make decisions for themselves.

The trait combination of dissociality and anankastia is not very common, but it can lead to horror stories such as that of Josef Fritzl, who in 1984 locked up his daughter, then only 18, in a sound-proofed basement of his house. Over the next 24 years, he repeatedly raped her and fathered seven children with her, one of whom died. It was only when his daughter managed to escape from the house that the full story came to light. Josef's wife, Rosemarie, who was on the floor above, never realised what was happening below. Although some find this surprising, the obsessional care with which her husband organised everything in the household and the degree of control he had over her meant she remained in total ignorance. Three of the children who were born of his rapes were adopted by the family as Josef was able to persuade Rosemarie they were foundlings.

This is an extreme example, but evidence that degrees of much less severe obsessional control is being exposed everywhere in families where domestic violence is present. Actual violence may not occur, as the pattern of behaviour that is used to gain or maintain power and control over anyone in a relationship can be carried out by implied threat only, but the figures suggest that across the world, and also in those with mental illness, nearly one in three of the population has experienced domestic violence (Oram et al., 2013; Sardinha et al., 2022).

This is not just a problem of personality. It is also deeply imbued with culture, and in some communities, particularly those with repressive regimes where women are relegated to servitude such as Afghanistan, it is likely to be higher. Adapting in this context is very difficult, not least as there is often no wish to adapt, and in this area, others may have to take on the task of correcting it.

Lifestyle and occupation

Work is therapeutic, and for the obsessional, it is curative. So whenever something goes wrong in life for the anankastic personality, the motto becomes similar to that of Boxer, the fictional horse in George Orwell's *Animal Farm*, who responds to every message about crops failing, disastrous weather, and turmoil, by saying, 'I will work harder'. The dangers are obvious. Work-life balance becomes completely disrupted, sleep is affected, exercise stops, and health problems mount.

It is possible with a few sharp reminders to get this balance back on track again. The simple question 'Are you happy with your life at present?' is unlikely to be answered positively once work has taken over disproportionately, and a correction can be made.

Leisure pursuits and conflict avoidance

Sport, games, and all competitions can preoccupy the obsessional mind as much as work, especially when the performance achieved is close to excellence. Excessive practice, rehearsal, and repetition can take over in the pursuit of betterment. In these situations, it is better if the leisure activity chosen is one in which the person does not excel, so it can be carried out with enthusiasm within a family framework, knowing that the outcome is completely unimportant.

References

Graham EK, Rutsohn JP, Turiano NA, Bendayan R, Batterham PJ, Gerstorf D, et al. (2017). Personality predicts mortality risk: an integrative data analysis of 15 international longitudinal studies. *Journal of Research in Personality*, 70, 174–186.

Oram S, Trevillion K, Feder G, & Howard LM (2013). Prevalence of experiences of domestic violence among psychiatric patients: systematic review. *British Journal of Psychiatry*, 202, 94–99.

Orwell G (1945). *Animal Farm*. Faber & Faber.

Sardinha L, Maheu-Giroux M, Stöckl H, Meyer SR, & García-Moreno C (2022). Global, regional, and national prevalence estimates of physical or sexual, or both, intimate partner violence against women in 2018. *Lancet*, 399, 803–813.

Chapter 14

Adaptation in practice

In this chapter, I am now assuming good knowledge of the nature of personality disturbance in terms of severity and domains and also the principles of nidotherapy. A road map is needed to put this into practice. Here it is, developed in four stages, both for those who feel they have personality problems at present and also for those who are wanting or being asked to help them.

The map has to trace adaptation in occupation, accommodation, and family relationships and social activities, and each can be examined in terms of the ICD-11 categories and trait domains.

Occupation

All occupation, whether paid or unpaid, is a boost to self-esteem provided it is chosen and not forced. There is a measure called a person-environment fit (P-E fit) (Caplan, 1987) that is a useful way of determining if a person is fitting in well or badly in their work. This can be measured in three ways:

> (a) the atomistic method, which examines perceptions of the person and environment as separate entities; (b) the molecular one, which concerns the perceived comparison between the person and environment; and (c) the molar method, which focuses on the subjectively perceived similarity, match, or fit between the person and environment (Edwards et al., 2006). These authors could have substituted 'personality' for 'person' in the last of these approaches, which is the best one for achieving a really harmonious match from the point of view of the subject, which is the central purpose of nidotherapy. A combination of the molar approach (subjective perception) and the atomistic approach (objective measurements) has been shown to lead to better satisfaction and performance.
>
> (Kühner et al., 2024)

DOI: 10.4324/9781003560630-14

Levels of personality disorder and occupation

Those with severe personality disorder are rarely involved in paid employment, so the luxury of choice is not often available. But some sort of occupational activity is always desirable. One of my patients who was originally seen as a homeless man in central London, where I was involved in a service for this population, became much more confident and also financially solvent by selling copies of *The Big Issue* outside Notting Hill Gate underground station (a very good perch) and later became a writer. If no paid work is available, then there are dozens of options as a volunteer.

For those with personality difficulty, there is a great deal of choice. It is just necessary to identify the aspects of the job that bring out the personality disturbance and find a way of either eliminating the aggravating ones or moving sideways to a different post. For those with mild and moderate personality disorder, the decision is more difficult and depends on the domain structure of the personality.

Occupation and the negative affective domain

The cardinal features of anxiety, worry, and need for safety dominate occupational choice for those with negative affectivity. For such people, the primary aim in an occupation is to feel comfortable, supported, and, at least to some extent, dependent, so there is always somebody you can rely on in times of difficulty. This can be achieved rather better in two types of organisation: ones which are very large and can accommodate many different types of people and others which are small and have very few employees, sometimes consisting of family members only, in which the job requirements are fashioned to suit the person and his or her personality.

Occupation and the detachment domain

Those who are independent and detached can prosper in occupational environments that others would cavil at or avoid. Many posts that are isolated and seem to be very boring are embraced with enthusiasm by someone who wishes are to be left alone and allowed to work independently.

Joel Paris gives a very good example of this in his book *Social Factors in the Personality Disorders*:

A 30-year-old paediatric nurse was referred by her supervisor because she was unable to manage the psychosocial aspects of her work. She was having particular difficulty with the deeds of the parents of hospitalized children. Her past history was that she had been unusually shy child would never formed meaningful relationships with her peers.

Her family was large, and her parents were too preoccupied to provide her with much individual attention since she was unusually bright she devoted herself to her studies. Adult she had no experience at all with the opposite sex. She did not feel deprived by her life choices. She was entirely devoted to her profession in which he was highly knowledgeable.

Dr Paris initiated a treatment we would now include as a component of nidotherapy.

A weekly series of psychotherapy sessions was instituted and lasted for six months. Overtly, the treatment seemed to lack any degree of content. The patient made little eye contact and was silent for long periods.

Over time she began to talk about her difficulties. In particular she was able to discuss how frightened she felt that the parents of the children she was treating would judge her harshly. At follow-up she was functioning much better at work. She had begun to work in the Arctic, where there was a great need for her services. She was more comfortable working in this alien culture, into which he would not in any case expect to fit she launched a successful career by developing services to the native populations there. She continued neither to desire nor to seek close relationships.

(Paris, 1996, pp. 175–176)

It is easy to see how this bright and committed nurse who had such problems in relationships with her peers would blossom in such an alien environment where past social fears could be tossed away.

Occupation and the detachment domain

Many of those with impulsive personalities move from one job to another in search of more stimulation and rapid reward. It is preferable to find an occupation where there is the opportunity for repeated highs and not too many lows, such as the entertainment industry with all its twists and turns, or life in a fashion house or a large sporting organisation. A life with good occupational excitement can prevent the search for more risky endeavours elsewhere. Another possibility is to have two or more part-time posts, at least one of which gives the right level of stimulation.

Occupation and the dissocial domain

It is often difficult to persuade those who have gained most of their assets from criminal activity that it is possible to be similarly successful by honest endeavour. 'If you think that, you're a sucker' is the instant response. But therapists have persevered. The Good Lives Model points out that what they call primary human goods include knowledge, excellence in both work and play, good relationships, spirituality, and creativity, and all are attempting to gain these. The model argues that when people offend in this pursuit, they are held up by their internal and external deficits. The carrots of this approach are much better than the sticks of punishment, and there is some evidence from case studies that when dissocial people are willing to consider change and well-trained therapists are administering this approach, there are positive outcomes (Barnao et al., 2016). But this is very weak evidence, and it comes from prisoners in correction centres, not people actively seeking treatment, and this critical distinction, discussed in Chapter 11, needs stressing. In nidotherapy, the therapist guides the person toward an occupation of the subject's choice; finding one that is not just a quick fix is a stiff challenge.

Occupation and the anankastic domain

One of the features of the anankastic personality is an excessive preoccupation with work, so one might imagine that nidotherapy might be easier in this population. There is no doubt that a degree of obsessionality is an excellent guide to work performance, but it is also true that this performance can become wildly awry when there is conflict between the perfectionistic standards of one person and the more easy-going attitudes of others. It is also sometimes necessary to suggest that an overworked and keen employee actually reduces their work hours rather than working far beyond them.

This is where an environmental advocate at work can come in useful. Occupational mental health is now becoming a subject of greater importance. It has long included advice on job placement, supervision after illness, and health counselling (Tyrer, 1987) but now is increasingly asking for those with experience in mental health nursing to apply for positions, and such applicants are likely to receive preference. If people are in doubt about the person-environmental fit, it is often the occupational health nurse who will be in the best position to advise.

Accommodation and the negative affective domain

Because the anxious person with strong negative affectivity is always in need of a place of safety, accommodation has a high priority. Personal circumstances and finances determine most aspects of accommodation, but the bare minimum for a fearful, nervous subject is the security of the premises, wherever it may be. The origin of the word 'nidotherapy' is the Latin *nidus*, the nest, as it conveys the impression of comfort, safety, and homeliness, expressed in German as *gemütlichkeit*, which wraps the concept up well in a cosy expression of welcoming warmth and belonging.

The attraction of the homely nest has in it the seeds of a problem. If the home is the only place where you feel calm and secure, you may not want to leave it too often, or, worse still, you may not want to leave it at all. Once you stay for long periods in the safety of home, all other places have the tendency to become more threatening, so agoraphobia develops, the fear of going to a threatening place outside, which is often associated with panic attacks and other episodes of high anxiety. This used to be called the syndrome of the housebound housewife, but it is no respecter of gender.

In Japan, there is a disorder called *hikikomori*. This is derived from the compound verb *hikikomoru*, that combines 'to pull back' (*hiku*) and 'to seclude oneself' (*komoru*). *Hikikomori* is a form of pathological social withdrawal or social isolation whose essential feature is physical isolation in one's home. It has been defined more precisely by Kato et al. (2019), but essentially, it is a combination of marked social isolation in one's home for at least six months, associated with significant functional impairment or distress. It is also associated with avoidant personality characteristics, and this fits in with negative affectivity. The age at onset is most often in adolescence or early adult life. It is estimated to affect 1.2% of the Japanese population (Koyama et al., 2010), with men comprising three-quarters of sufferers, with a lower proportion in other nations (Nonaka et al., 2022). These are very high figures and explain the concern many have with this condition, particularly as it takes males away from productive occupations at an important part of their lives.

In adapting to a more normal lifestyle, there needs to be an accommodating framework in which some regular activities take place outside the home. These need not be work related and should be enjoyable and desired. Eventually, these need to be linked to some sort of employment.

Accommodation and the detached domain

Preoccupation with staying at home and reluctance to venture elsewhere are not confined to negative affectivity. Detached personalities are happier when alone and have no problems in spending most of their lives in isolation if there is no outside stimulation or necessity to leave the home. The difference between those with detachment and those with negative affectivity is that those who are just detached have no fears out of doors; they are just disinterested.

Hikikomori in a detached personality has been successfully treated with nidotherapy in one published description. Sakamoto et al. (2005) describe a man with the condition in Oman who was unsuccessful in finding a job and gradually drifted further into reclusiveness. He had no desire to be close to his nuclear or extended family, preferring to spend his time in his own room and to be left alone undisturbed. The detailed account suggests strong elements of detachment.

> The father often knocked on his door to scold him for being lazy and to condemn him for not praying or doing something meaningful for himself. He told us that he preferred staying in the dark. He slept during the day time and stayed awake at night watching satellite television or playing video games. Food was left at his door and he returned the trays when finished. When family members were away during working hours or at sleep at night, he was noted to tiptoe into the kitchen to replenish his supplies for his room.
>
> During our meetings with him, SD complained that his family had taken him to various hospitals in Oman and nearby countries to get him 'treated', which he strongly disliked.

The adaptive policy of nidotherapy was then tried successfully.

> Rather than adopting a hostile attitude toward him, the family was encouraged to be accommodating and reduce their caustic tone whenever they encountered him in the house. The father stopped knocking on his door to wake him up. When family members reduced their criticisms of him, he began to selectively socialise with some of them. Occasionally he agreed to venture with a family member out for a drive, picnic, or dining out. In the last year, when a job vacancy opened that entailed only evening shifts, he agreed to work. His evening shift had minimal interaction with other people. On our last contact with the family, seven years after he had developed reclusive behavior and two years after being brought in for psychiatric consultation, he remains well and now has been given a full-time job at his workplace.
>
> (Sakamoto et al., 2005, pp. 193–194)

The authors explained the success of nidotherapy as accommodating to his behaviour more successfully, ceasing to put conditions on it and appreciating his wishes. As a consequence,

> [H]e became less antagonist and more social, which, in turn, reduced his distress and suffering and improved functioning. When the family members adopted a stance of accommodating his reclusive interpersonal functioning, his distress that made him resort to his reclusive lifestyle gradually abated and he returned to full-time work.
>
> (Sakamoto et al., 2005, p. 194)

Once more attractive alternatives outside the home are available to the detached person (e.g., fixed social occasions such as chess where all the rules are clear, bird-watching, plant identification), they are readily taken up with no anxiety.

Accommodation and the disinhibited domain

There is a tendency for disinhibited people to move around from one type of accommodation to another, and very few places are treasured or revered. The need to put a personal stamp on any habitation may lead to curious architectural changes that may not always impress the neighbours or satisfy the needs of the person concerned. A place that is loved and adored at first can quickly become a rejected disaster, so it is always valuable to have a moderating individual to prevent mistakes and excesses. A wise counsel is often what is needed in advance of otherwise rash decisions.

Accommodation and the dissocial domain

Dissociality shows itself in different ways depending on the background of the individuals concerned. There are some situations that are highly profitable for the get-rich-quick entrepreneurs with well-honed antennae: 'rapid business growth, increased downsizing, frequent reorganisations, mergers, acquisitions, and joint ventures have inadvertently increased the number of attractive employment opportunities for individuals with psychopathic personalities' (Babiak, 2007). Once successful, the accommodation of such people approaches Mar-a-Lago proportions with opulence glowing from every corner. At the opposite extreme, the repeated recidivist lives in squalor in run-down hostels or even on the street, with no interest apart from staying dry and warm. It is very difficult to give advice consistent with nidotherapy here as it is unlikely to be followed, and unfortunately, if it is desired strongly by the persuasive patient, it may be disastrous to the therapist.

Accommodation and the anankastic domain

In my experience, one of the best ways of assessing anankastia is to make a home visit. Apart from having to take your shoes off at the front door, you will have to be careful not to disturb any ornaments no matter where placed in the rooms, any alteration to the symmetry of chairs around the tables must be carefully resisted, and avoid going to the toilet unless you absolutely have to, because something is bound to go wrong. I exaggerate a little, but I have also learnt in nidotherapy not to interfere with this degree of order. It is only when it becomes time consuming and out of control that some intervention is required. But you have to wait for this to be asked for; do not offend by diving in and trying to alter a treasured obsession. It is when anankastia slows every venture down to a snail's pace that gentle advice may be needed. As much as possible, simple solutions should outweigh complex ones.

In addition to moving to a new environment to suit your needs, there is also the possibility of staying where you are and adjusting the environment to suit you. This option can be very favourable. Here is an example from my recent experience. A farmer with a large family was concerned about his family's occupational future after his death. He realised that not many of his three sons and two daughters would want to continue farming. He hit on an ingenious solution. He organised the division of his land into five roughly equal plots. He gave each of his children one of these plots and left the decision about the use of the land to each child. But to maintain the cohesion of the family, he made it a legal requirement that if any of the children sold their plots, the proceeds would be returned to the family, and they would get no personal gain. This arrangement would only work if all the family agreed to it. They did so wholeheartedly. Sadly, the farmer has now died, but his legacy continues. All his family members live in the same site, they have many different occupations, and none of them have continued farming, but each has used their land well and are making a good living. In the language of *Alice in Wonderland*, 'everyone has won and all shall have prizes'.

Family and social relationships

Family relationships and levels of personality disturbance

The definition of personality disorder includes all aspects of family relationships. In severe personality disorder, they are close to non-existent—'family relationships are absent (despite having living relatives) or marred by significant conflict'—and even in mild personality disorder, there are difficulties that are less but still significant 'either limited to circumscribed areas (e.g. romantic relationships; employment) or present in more areas but of milder severity'. But families, despite amazing difficulties, still have a tendency to stick together. In assessing someone with significant personality problems, particularly when they appear to be completely devoid of friends, look for a compassionate family member; one can often be found. Once the right person is identified, the abyss that previously separated the individual from society can be bridged. One of our patients was in a state of almost constant conflict with her neighbours, the staff in the nearby café where she was repeatedly banned for bad behaviour, and the mental health service where her rudeness was considered so offensive she was almost excluded from care. But when her fortunes seemed to have hit rock bottom, a former boy-friend returned and befriended her, and subsequently, they married. Her anger softened, she regained her sense of humour, and the change was noted by all.

Family relationships and negative affectivity

The main consequence of negative affectivity in families is the development of unhelpful close relationships. Because the nervous person is reluctant to embrace any form of change, other family members have to set aside time and effort in extra support. This can develop into passive resignation—not a satisfactory outcome—or, if tackled more constructively, provide a supportive environment from others. Many families who are reluctant to place their elderly relatives in care homes are often pleasantly surprised by the positive reaction to a new environment that is safe, provides an active social life with very little personal responsibility or worry, and is much more stimulating than the previous one at home. But it does not necessarily require a care home for that purpose; families can help add extras to these lives in many ways.

Family relationships and detachment

Those who are detached often have poor relationships with their families, but this need not be so. If a lifeline exists between the person and the family that is activated regularly, it can be an ideal way of maintaining communication. An annual get-together, a team game, a quiz night, and involvement in a joint competition all can bring the detached person back into the fold. But the subject chosen has to be one that is embraced with enthusiasm by everybody, and although detached people often have single-person interests, they are rarely exclusive.

Family relationships and disinhibition

It is often difficult for families to stay in regular touch with their more impulsive and reckless members, but in this age of the internet, it is now much easier. If the only occasions when contact is made is when problems arise from an impulsive act, then families are none too pleased. Channels of communication should always be kept open, often with a key family member with immense patience and tolerance.

Family relationships and dissociality

The problems arising from dissociality often involve family separation and sometimes the past histories of those who have suffered trauma and abuse lead to a complete absence of family connections. Imprisonment also separates people from families, but the maintenance of contact during a prison sentence and the support that is needed afterward are often key to successful rehabilitation.

Family relationships and anankastia

Anankastic personalities need solid supporting relationships for the most part as these add security. Sometimes the best relationships are achieved when there is no competition involved. A person with a drive to strong achievement may find it difficult to get a good relationship with a peer, but when a young or older person is in support, the element of competition does not arise.

Colleagues at work can also act in the same way for such personalities as family members. They can provide the additional understanding from knowledge of the nature of the person's work that would be only vaguely known to a family member.

References

Babiak P (2007). *Snakes in Suits: When Psychopaths Go to Work*. Harper-Collins.

Barnao M, Ward T, & Casey S (2016). Taking the good life to the institution: forensic service users' perceptions of the good lives model. *International Journal of Offender Therapy and Comparative Criminology*, 60, 766–786.

Caplan RD (1987). Person-environment fit theory and organizations: commensurate dimensions, time perspectives, and mechanisms. *Journal of Vocational Behavior*, 31, 248–267.

Edwards JR, Cable DM, Williamson IO, Lambert LS, & Shipp AJ (2006). The phenomenology of fit: linking the person and environment to the subjective experience of person-environment fit. *Journal of Applied Psychology*, 91, 802–827.

Kato TA, Kanba S, & Teo AR (2019). Hikikomori: multidimensional understanding, assessment, and future international perspectives. *Psychiatry & Clinical Neuroscience*, 73, 427–440.

Koyama A, Miyake Y, Kawakami N, Tsuchiya M, Tachimori H, & Takeshima T; World Mental Health Japan Survey Group (2010). Lifetime prevalence, psychiatric comorbidity and demographic correlates of "hikikomori" in a community population in Japan. *Psychiatry Research*, 176, 69–74.

Kühner C, Stein M, & Zacher H (2024). A Person-Environment Fit approach to environmental sustainability in the workplace. *Journal of Environmental Psychology*, 95, 102270.

Nonaka S, Takeda T, & Sakai M (2022). Who are hikikomori? demographic and clinical features of hikikomori (prolonged social withdrawal): a systematic review. *Australian and New Zealand Journal of Psychiatry*, 56, 1542–1554.

Paris J (1996). *Social Factors in the Personality Disorders: A Biopsychosocial Approach to Etiology and Treatment*. Cambridge University Press.

Sakamoto N, Martin RG, Kumano H, Kuboki T, & Al-Adawi S (2005). Hikikomori, is it a culture-reactive or culture-bound syndrome? nidotherapy and a clinical vignette from Oman. *International Journal of Psychiatry in Medicine*, 35, 191–198.

Tyrer F (1987). Organization of occupational health services. In: JK Howard & F Tyrer (eds.), *Textbook of Occupational Medicine*, pp. 21–45. Oxford University Press.

Chapter 15

Adapting nidotherapy to mental health services

Nidotherapy is both a principle and a strategy of management, so it can readily be adapted to mental health services as well as individuals, and in some places, this is already happening. But it has far to go. The whole structure needs major reform, not fiddling at the edges, and, sadly, many of the changes that have been introduced in recent years have contradicted all the principles of nidotherapy and good practice. Massive reduction in psychiatric beds, far greater in the UK than every other developed country (Tyrer, 2024), lies behind many of these changes.

Inpatient services

Here is one example that illustrates the complete failure of the modern NHS to understand the needs of patients. The change is better described by Ballatt & Campling in their book *Intelligent Kindness* (2011), which reflected the original aim of the NHS in emphasising 'the importance of kinship, compassion and mutual support', qualities that comprised the essential oil that lubricated the early years of the NHS. But the system that exists now is divisive, uncompassionate, and flawed. It forgets the essentials and ticks pointless targets instead. Here is one example that shows the system is completely alien to the principles of nidotherapy.

Before I retired from NHS practice, I worked in an assertive outreach team which tried as much as possible to treat patients in the community without ever admitting them to hospital. But when they needed to be admitted, I looked after them as the team consultant together with my junior doctors and the inpatient nursing team. This combination allowed each inpatient stay to be as short as possible, and often, it could be planned in advance as a short admission for respite care. When, for example, a patient was in a crisis, was suicidal, disturbed, and unable to cope at home but from experience we knew it would be short-lived, we could ask for a respite admission. This is not a psychiatric emergency; it did not require a crisis team or a new major treatment, but it could be easily be managed by respite care.

DOI: 10.4324/9781003560630-15

Respite admissions rarely lasted for more than a few days, and the most important aspect was that continuity of care was maintained. The phrase 'continuity of care' is repeated over and over by those who plan services but do not deliver them. Unfortunately, in recent years, continuity of care has become a hollow joke. The way the services are set up leads to severe fragmentation of care, not continuity. I felt I could not continue in the service once a new policy was introduced, without consultation, that all inpatient services would be separated from community ones. This meant the patients on admission were looked after by a completely new team headed by a new consultant. The time when a patient is admitted to hospital is often a very stressful and anxious one, and if you are presented on admission with a set of strange faces and an abundance of questions about your past life and current problems, you are not in the best position to be able to deal with them. When the team who has been looking after you already has a plan for your care, it is a complete waste of time start again with a new assessment by people who are complete strangers to you.

I campaigned against this new policy without much success. I am not a good campaigner when I am annoyed because my impulsive personality traits take over, and I say things I have to apologise for later. 'Utterly ridiculous' was a favourite one of mine. I rudely asked all who were involved to see the evidence in favour of this new system and found there was none. There was just a vague supposition that an inpatient team focused on rapid management might be able to get a patient out of hospital more quickly than a team whose key staff were based in the community, as they can be more focused on discharge. The thinking here is always the same; any form of management that can reduce the use of expensive inpatient beds should be embraced fully, irrespective of any other considerations. Patients' preferences go out of the window despite the standard mantra, 'we put patients first', which is trotted out endlessly.

This diktat from the Department of Health was the complete opposite of care with nidotherapy. Patients were not consulted about this change; there were no exceptions, and everyone had to follow the rules. All respite admissions ceased. Even the evidence that patients admitted under our team spent less than half the time in hospital that other consultants' admissions did had absolutely no impact. End of story. It was time for me to leave. Subsequent research showed that the policy was heavily disliked by patients, and in a comparison of five countries, those in the UK were less satisfied with their experiences of inpatient care than all others (Bird et al., 2020). Continuity of care is no longer practised by clinicians, yet when it is provided by others, such as peer-support workers, it has been found to be effective (Johnson et al., 2018). Perhaps this may jolt services into a rethink.

It is now virtually impossible to practise the skills of nidotherapy in current NHS inpatient units, mainly because the number of beds available for acute care is so limited and the pressures to discharge so great. I am a great believer in community care when it is practised in conjunction with an adequate number of beds as it then reduces admissions, improves satisfaction, and saves more lives than alternative approaches (Simmonds et al., 2001), and as almost all these patients would have personality disturbance with the ICD-11 diagnostic system, we can conclude that good community care is right for personality disordered patients also.

Case example

I now give an individual case example of someone we tried to help using nidotherapy, but we were foiled at every turn by a broken system. Elizabeth was a small Afro Caribbean lady who had a recurrent psychotic depressive illness and a very anxious personality. When her depression was very severe, she had to be admitted to hospital and sometimes had a course of electroconvulsive therapy (ECT), still the most powerful form of treatment for severe depression despite the awful publicity it tends to receive because its administration simply appears barbaric.

After we had treated her in hospital with ECT, she was discharged and initially made good progress. Unfortunately, there were family problems that precipitated another episode of depression, and I went to see her with a nurse from our team. She was sitting in an old coat in her flat on the third floor of a council building, telling us that recriminatory voices were saying she was useless, and there was no point in living.

'We are going to have to admit you to hospital again, Elizabeth', I said, knowing that her previous experiences of a highly disturbed, chaotic, noisy ward were very unpleasant ones.

'I'm not going back to that awful hell-hole again. All those men coming into the dormitory, shouting at the top of their voices; it's just too frightening. I'm very small; I can't defend myself. Can't I go somewhere else?'

'I agree, Elizabeth. The acute unit is not right for you, but we have no alternative since they closed down the rehabilitation unit close by just over a year ago. But if you come along with us now, we can get a full assessment of how you are and find some sort of answer. I cannot promise anything because we have so few places available for people to be treated in safe surroundings'.

We spent nearly half an hour trying to persuade her to come with us for this assessment. In the end, she agreed and came with us. Halfway down the iron steps running down to the ground, she suddenly stopped.

'Sorry, I can't go there again. I just can't'. She turned round and climbed back up the steps to the floor where she lived.

Shortly afterward, we returned to her flat after getting agreement for her to be assessed at our community base, which was not at the hospital.

We thought this would be a good compromise, but by now, she was completely fixed in her view. We explained our dilemma to her son, who also lived with her, and he sympathised but could not think of anything more we could do.

Two days later, we got a message from the son that his mother had hanged herself. Neither she nor we could find a way out of her mental prison apart from suicide.

In an attempt to compensate for this tragedy, I tried to persuade the hospital authorities to reopen the rehabilitation unit they had just closed. This would have been a much better place for Elizabeth to be assessed and treated, but it was no more. Not surprisingly, I failed in my plea.

All doctors fail at times, and when they do, it is easy to attribute blame. Henry Marsh, the neurosurgeon who has brilliantly exposed his professional life, often in excoriating detail, describes how he, at a relatively early point in his career, had to remove a very large brain tumour. The tumour was benign (i.e., would not spread to other parts of the body) but would go on growing if any was left behind at the operation. Henry described how the operation went, very well at first, and then at the end, he had tried to remove the last part, deep inside the brain, and cut an important artery, the basilar artery. This is the artery to the brain stem, the telephone system of life, and Henry knew that the patient would now never recover. Seven years later, the patient was alive but curled up on a bed unconscious with no life of any meaning. Henry, in his book *Do No Harm* (Marsh, 2014), called this chapter 'Hubris', but this was a little unfair. He had just failed at the last hurdle, the very last hurdle, and any surgeon could have done the same.

Psychiatrists do not usually face this do-or-die dilemma, but we often make mistakes, either through inaction or over-treatment with drugs, and deserve criticism when we do. But when you are part of a system that has failed, you are on a more difficult platform. You can rail and storm against the managers and the accountants and the politicians, but if you are part of that system, you also bear some responsibility. I felt I bore some responsibility for Elizabeth's death; I could have done more to alter the way the service was run. One of my close friends, Peter Carter, who was the chief executive of the trust where I worked in the 1990s, used to complain to me that clinicians who wanted their services should spend some of their time as managers instead of always sniping from the wings, and he was right. Peter listened to clinicians carefully, but this was not enough on its own. But I am sure he would not mind me repeating what he was asked by Gordon Brown, then Chancellor of the Exchequer, why his was the only trust in London not running at a loss. 'I listen to the clinicians', Peter answered, 'and when instructions come down from the Department of Health that they think are sensible, I adopt them; when they think they are silly, I ignore them'.

At this point, I will take on the role of manager and explain how, with nidotherapy and other approaches, we ought to change the system of care so it does genuinely put patients first, including those with personality disorders that many like to dismiss as being of no consequence. This takes us into the dynamic relationship between inpatient and community care.

A balanced equilibrium between hospital and community

'A reasonable starting point in planning mental health services is to provide them in relation to the *specific* needs of people with mental health problems in the local area', wrote Thornicroft and Tansella in 2006. Absolutely right, and exactly what the proponents of nidotherapy would say. Identify the needs by asking what they are, preferably linking the individual with area needs, and devote your resources accordingly.

But we don't start off with policies that address the specific needs of people who are mentally ill; we never have done. Some years ago, I interviewed Kenneth Clarke, former Chancellor of the Exchequer and, before that, Minister of Health, and he made an observation during that interview that struck home. 'You must realise', he said in his blokey voice,

> that politicians are primarily interested in votes. The trouble with you and your colleagues in mental health is that you do not have a large mental health lobby acting on your behalf. You ought to have, as you are much larger than the many other health organisations to whom we listen carefully. If we got to the point when mental health services might be disadvantaged by a policy and had to say 'we can't do that; it would upset the mental health lobby', then you could be sure you were having an impact. But we have never got to that point.

There is an important organisation, MIND, that began its life as the National Association of Mental Health and does valuable work in promoting mental health initiatives across the country. But the only time it had real major influence on health policy was when Kenneth Robinson, the first chair of MIND when it changed its name, became Minister of Health. He gave a very impressive talk to us as undergraduates at Cambridge University in 1959, when he outlined his vision for mental health services in the future. It was a marvellous vision, but it has never been properly realised.

If the mental health lobby is to have stronger influence, it probably needs to be politicised. The only place in the world where mental health patients have been properly listened to is Trieste in the north-east of Italy, whose voice was heard by Franco Basaglia when he came to a mental hospital just north of Trieste in Gorizia.

When Basaglia arrived at Gorizia in the 1960s, he was shocked by the standard institutional environment masquerading as care, with locked doors; a background of distressed people weeping and moaning; staff moving silently and hiding in the nursing stations, hardly knowing what to do; and a complete absence of therapeutic activity. (Just in case you think this was exceptional, the mental hospitals I worked in during the 1960s in England had 'back wards' that were exactly the same.)

Basaglia blamed the culture of the institution for this travesty of care. It had already been described by Russell Barton as institutional neurosis, 'a disease characterized by apathy, lack of initiative, loss of interest in things and events not immediately personal or present, submissiveness, and sometimes no expression of feelings of resentment at harsh or unfair orders' (Barton, 1959). Basaglia started his process of reform in 1961. He stopped the practice of binding patients to their beds, abolished the isolation of patients in separate rooms, and started a debate about the use of mental hospitals all over Italy. This led to the passing of a national reform bill in 1978 that led to the closure of mental hospitals countrywide. The main consequence of institutional care was the suppression of the patient's voice; after the enlightened views of the early reformers, who set up mental hospitals in the verdant countryside where their talents could blossom, the views of patients were squeezed remorselessly into silence.

With mental health reform, their voices came back, and they celebrated with local communities as bonfires were lit to mark hospital closures. I was present at one of the last closures in 2003, at Montelupo just south of Florence, when the last forensic institution based in one of the finest Medici villas was closed. It was a celebration masquerading as an international meeting. Speeches were given at first in the deadpan and boring tones of pseudoscience; then the speakers were interrupted by shouts from the last group of penitentiary patients who then milled into the conference room and herded all outside where a bright blue papier-mâché horse with the most enormous buttocks towed a large sleepy beast of uncertain parentage and poor dentition, the dragon of Montelupo, toward the main gates of the penitentiary. The gates were raised, and the townspeople waiting on the other side cheered wildly as a brass band accompanied the throng to the market square, where a short but impassioned speech concluded the closure of the hospital: 'All forensic psychiatric hospitals should be closed; they do not prevent violence; they only reproduce it'.

Some have decried what has been called 'the Italian experience' and claimed it has just transferred institutional care to community neglect, but the overall effect has been to support the Thornicroft and Tansella aim of addressing and satisfying the 'specific needs of people with mental health problems in the local area'. The former locked institutions are now open and filled with patients' activities—local broadcasts, café chatter, a debating place, a sewing room where clothing is being made. One important aspect of the Trieste reform was to offer work opportunities to discharged patients, a very important environmental aim that we come across frequently in nidotherapy. There are few things more important to someone's self-esteem than the knowledge that they are part of society and doing something useful.

Although the Trieste approach would be unlikely to work in the same way in the United Kingdom—we are too buttoned up as a nation—the system can be reformed using the same principles. The combination of listening to concerns, assessment of needs, changes in the environment to match these needs, and a ready response to changing circumstances are all components of nidotherapy that work toward better health. 'We do not have enough resources' is a frequent plaintive lament, but it is over-used. There are too many middle managers in the NHS. Basaglia did not need so many when he reformed the Trieste services, and many tore up the rule book and helped in implementing the reforms.

Those with personality problems also have a role here. Note that most inpatients in all centres have some degree of personality dysfunction, and sometimes they are not the best at creating a common front with others. But they also have strengths, and these can come in useful in difficult negotiations. Persistent use of a battering ram will break down any door, and sticky people can often stick with a plan longer than most others.

A vision of a new adapted service

First referral

If we combine all the positives we know about providing better mental health services, we have a template for a new system. I outline this next.

Patients are referred to the service by general practitioners and other health professionals. A patient can also make a self-referral that is screened before an appointment is made. Assessments are made by either a single practitioner or a small team. Any assessments made without the patient being present need to be short and time limited; they should not be used as a filter to refer to other services unless the request is considered inappropriate, and this is agreed unequivocally.

Care is provided for patients who are accepted for treatment after a full assessment which also includes one of personality status. If drug treatment is prescribed, it should be discussed fully and only implemented after full agreement with the patient in a genuinely collaborative way (Tyrer, 2024). Patients are consulted about the ways they hope to be treated. Any views they have should be treated with respect and, if they are not followed, a full explanation given. At the end of the interview, the patient should have a good idea what exactly is wrong with them, whether it needs specific treatment, and, if so, for how long and also have some idea of the likely prognosis. If continued care is required, then a care coordinator will ensure continuity.

If the patient needs a more specialised service (e.g., for eating disorder, stress-related conditions, psychosis), this should be given by the relevant personnel within the service. The treatment should not be hived off to another centre where there will be no further contact with the team. If you are in a small silo of practitioners seeing only one type of problem, you are going to promote burn-out; we all need some variety. In any case, so many patients have conditions which could require input from several different services, and it has to be well coordinated within the service to avoid confusion. The practice of referring from one team to another should be avoided wherever possible. General practitioners should be informed about decisions made.

Continued outpatient care

Continued care should be a joint process between the psychiatric team and primary care. At times it may be appropriate for the psychiatric team to be seeing the patient in primary care facilities in order to improve liaison. The current practice, far too frequently followed, of just discharging a patient from psychiatric care with no clear instructions about follow-up or continuation of medication should be avoided. Patients' views about continued care and where it should take place should always be listened to carefully and followed wherever possible.

Inpatient care

The hospital environment should be regarded as an extension of community care. Staff who work in the hospital should also have responsibilities in the community so they can be reassured about the nature of and input necessary for good community care. This can ensure a smooth transition following discharge. The immediate period after discharge is a very sensitive time and as much as possible needs to be made smooth and undramatic. Sudden discharge to make a bed available should be avoided wherever possible.

Patients should have a say in the construction of inpatient units; at present they are largely ignored. Whilst there is no wish to go back to the days of large, spacious mental hospitals where the main therapy appeared to be a better environment than the patients' previous ones, there were advantages in the extra space and privacy. Vincent van Gogh's artistic output was at its greatest when he was an inpatient at Saint-Rémy-de-Provence mental hospital in 1889 where he stayed for a year as a voluntary patient. He would have had little time to paint had he been in a modern inpatient unit.

The responsibility for treatment and subsequent discharge from hospital should be made jointly by inpatient and community team staff. There is normally no need for consultants to work entirely within hospitals as in this environment, their community care skills would diminish, and their judgment would likely be ineffective. Transfer to other hospitals should be very rare. Before discharge, relevant members of the community team involved with the treatment of the patient should also be attending hospital reviews and giving opinions.

Transfer to rehabilitation and other services

If a patient is in hospital for more than three months, a review of continued care is necessary. All mental health services should have a rehabilitative component—this is often called a recovery component, but the meaning is the same—and this should include inpatient facilities. Most developed countries have a good range of rehabilitative services; currently, the United Kingdom does not have enough residential units.

Members of rehabilitation service should have regular contact with the community teams and may sometimes share responsibilities. This liaison is important if the patient is going to be transferred back to the community team after leaving rehabilitation. The relatives of the patient and others who will be subsequently involved with their care should also have regular contact with the rehabilitation services before any discharge is planned.

The development of rehabilitation teams may include access to new premises. Outpatient rehabilitation is being carried out very effectively by recovery colleges across the country, but this does not include inpatient care.

Because there has been great attention given to the new community initiatives in the last few years, the importance of inpatient facilities has been neglected. The need for inpatient care has sometimes been labelled a failure of care, but this is nonsense. The process of care can be regarded as a set of building blocks, of which inpatient care is a most important part. The process of this building has to be a joint one in which each phase adds to what has previously been achieved. Far too often, an inpatient admission fails to be part of the rehabilitation process, and clinical teams feel they have to start from scratch again. This can only succeed if the inpatient services regard themselves as integral to the whole team.

Many years ago, I compared an ideal mental health system to the beehive. Each community area, ideally a hexagon as in the beehive combs, would serve the whole population in that area. The community outreach staff, like the worker bees, would identify the areas where mental illness was most pronounced. They would then come back to the community base or hospital and ensure that more resources were deployed to those areas. This would ensure that those with the greatest need received the most care (Tyrer, 1985). If this was followed with the same diligence shown by the bees, those in the most deprived areas would receive the most care and so contradict the inverse care law of the well-known GP Julian Tudor Hart: '[T]he availability of good medical care tends to vary inversely with the need for it in the population served' (Hart, 1971). Unfortunately, across the world, the inverse care law is still true.

Social prescribing, the additional facility of referral to a link worker to ensure that the social environment fits the requirements of the patient, has links to nidotherapy but is still at a very primitive state (Tyrer & Boardman, 2020). In a full systematic independent review, the state of the intervention was baldly exposed in the summary: '[T]here is an absence of evidence for social prescribing link workers' (Kiely et al., 2022). This is not surprising as the intervention is poorly defined, does not involve trained health personnel, and has uncertain defined outcomes. We would like it to be combined with nidotherapy to make it effective and also extend it to the people who would particularly benefit (Poole & Huxley, 2024).

Discharge after a prolonged hospital admission

An important component of a comprehensive mental health service is to provide all the necessary support for those who have been discharged from hospital after a long admission. Exactly the same difficulty is found when prisoners are released after a long sentence; so many of them are completely rudderless and have nowhere to turn.

But there are effective ways of making this important step a smooth transition. Horton Rehabilitation Services in Surrey are well placed to carry out successful discharge as they have managed to retain their original hospital site covering five acres. Many of the patients who have been transferred there have had hospital admissions lasting several years, and all the dangers of institutionalisation are present. Horton is now practising nidotherapy to help successful discharge in the same way that our original trial practised nidotherapy (Ranger et al., 2009). When patients are approaching the time for discharge, they are moved to smaller cottages at the edge of the site where they have less supervision and are able to carry out activities of daily living such as cooking and caring for themselves. All have clear ideas of where they would like to go after leaving hospital, and, as much as possible, these take into account and plan the discharge arrangements.

Special attention is paid to the social environment as well as the physical one, and patients have the opportunity of visiting places and, in some

cases, having a test period of living in the accommodation before a decision is reached about discharge. Because the service is not under pressure
to admit new patients, there is rarely a need to set a deadline unless one
is determined by the patient or other influences. As a consequence of this
careful approach, very few of the discharges fail.

My criticisms of current services are not just isolated stormings in a wilderness. A large number of my colleagues feel exactly the same way and,
unfortunately, most commonly react by retiring early and spending their
lives in what they judge to be more productive enterprises. At the simplest
level, the training we all have received should provide us with the ability
to help patients at difficult points in their lives, but the system of care we
now encounter contradicts all our training. We are no longer caring for our
patients; we are processing them.

One of my colleagues, Martin Deahl, puts it bluntly:

> Medicine, and especially psychiatry, should be led by professionals who
> put the patient, not the bottom line, first. Psychiatry's raison d'être is
> to protect the interests of some of society's most vulnerable individu-
> als, and attempt to recreate a working environment that allows for the
> return of a fulfilled, rewarding, professional career. Failing to protect
> our interests and restore some of our professional esteem ultimately lets
> our patients, as well as ourselves down, and may well be signalling the
> end of psychiatry as we know it.
>
> (Deahl, 2024)

The suggestions made in this chapter are not going to be adopted overnight, if ever. Others might ask what a chapter like this is doing in a book
on adapting to the symptoms of personality disorder. I maintain that it
is completely apposite. The patients who require the most therapeutic of
relationships are those with personality problems. If you have had a brief
episode of depression and are treated with antidepressants successfully, the
therapeutic relationship almost becomes a luxury additive. It is good to
have it, but it is not essential. Those with personality problems, and I need
to repeat again that these are the people who dominate the referrals to
mental health care, need to have good, steady relationships to negotiate the
ups and downs of their passage through difficult times. When one of my
patients was in a productive partnership with a therapist she trusted and
then, unexpectedly, was told by the therapist that she had been moved to a
different area, she asked, not unreasonably, if she could still continue seeing her. The famous cartoonist H. M. Bateman had a side-splitting series
showing the impact of social gaffes in stuffy 20th-century Britain, called
'The Man Who'. Nowadays, in today's mental health services, these would
be a little more likely to address 'The Woman Who', and the one that

would lead to hollow laughter across the vistas of NHS psychiatry would be 'the patient who asked to continue with the same therapist'.

One approach that has been adopted across the NHS in the UK is to place patients on pathways of care. The notion of this appears at first to be a good one. People with common conditions such as eating or bipolar disorders have similar needs and can be treated together. But everyone recognises that there is a tremendous amount of overlap between these conditions. It is commonly called comorbidity, but this term, which means two separate disorders existing in the same person, is very rarely true as the conditions are not genuinely separate. I have been asked on several occasions to advise on the 'personality disorder pathway'. I have always answered that the personality pathway should be universal; it applies to all, cannot be separated, and to place people in such a pathway is stigmatising and counter-productive.

It is perfectly possible for mental health services to adapt, even at a time of financial restriction, a circumstance that is now so common it is hardly worth saying. The mental health lobby could ensure their concerns went straight to the top, provided the lobby was large enough to force the system to change. When professionals working in services complain collectively, there is always the riposte that they are looking after their own interests and not those of others. This can never be used against patients, who can reply, 'Yes, indeed, we are looking after our interests, and they are meant to be yours as well'.

In an ideal scenario, each community would have responsibilities to maintain mental health in its area. It would have a say in where inpatient provision would be placed, would help in placing people after leaving hospital, and, perhaps most importantly, identify mental health problems before they got out of hand. This would not be a formal requirement, but if communities were genuinely able to understand their residents and be sensitive to change, then what I am writing would appear commonplace.

Currently, our charity, NIDUS-UK, is carrying out a study in several villages in the county of Nottinghamshire. The villages are small, most of the inhabitants are relatively affluent, and the rate of severe mental illness is likely to be low. But because the population is relatively stable, it offers the opportunity the study changes over time, including environmental changes that are carried out as a consequence of nidotherapy. Many of the environmental changes planned are communal ones that affect the whole community. We are looking to see if these villages can come together and work in harmony so mental health is preserved and enhanced, both in the shorter and longer term.

This project comes into the realm of preventive psychiatry, a part of the subject that is grossly ignored by conventional research and service evaluation. Our project includes a cost-effectiveness analysis (Tyrer et al.,

2025), and we expect that the nidotherapy intervention will be particularly valuable here as it will be mainly preventive and cost little. Whether this will have any impact on service provision is quite another matter, and the general attitudes toward initiatives of this nature are not encouraging:

> [L]ack of awareness of the substantial economic savings from preventive interventions for mental disorders, the need for an initial investment in training and investment of time by professionals (often with no short-term return), and stigma, partly explain the lower interest in mental health prevention than in other areas of medicine. It might take more time to realise the benefits of investing in prevention for mental health than in other areas of medicine (e.g., oncology or cardiovascular disease), which is problematic when politicians need to prioritise their health actions on the basis of what can be communicated to future voters in 4–5-year election cycles.
>
> (Arango et al., 2018, p. 596)

The physical environment in mental health services

The changes in psychiatric architecture in recent years have been diabolical to good mental health. Unfortunately, despite much sensible guidance being given to the process of inpatient admission, care, and discharge by successive editions of the Royal College of Psychiatrists' College Centre for Quality Improvement (CCQI), there is no mention of the required architecture of these settings. The closure of mental hospitals with their abundant grounds was followed by relocation to inpatient units, frequently squeezed into the remaining unwanted corners of general hospitals, with poor natural lighting, difficulty in access, and limited space for any form of leisure activity (the patients in one unit in central London have their exercise area in a cage on the roof), and often, no outdoor space. These units are often placed in inner city locations and make no attempt to suppress external noise, have few facilities for joint meetings of patients and their relatives, and increasingly resemble new versions of Jeremy Bentham's 18th-century panopticons.

It is worth giving a description of these structures as they represent an excellent example of Bentham's philosophy of utilitarianism, a monstrosity of a noun but one that followed the principle that happiness and well-being were the main aims of life. Panopticons were set in prisons and comprised two circular towers, one inside the other, the outer one containing cells that faced the inner tower. The guards in this tower would be invisible to prisoners but would have an unobstructed view of each cell. This would allegedly lead to happiness in both parties as the guards could offer oversight without difficulty, and the inmates could rest in what Bentham described as 'a sequestered and observed solitude' (Bentham, 1791).

Because of the obsession with risk dominating psychiatric services, we are gradually moving toward the principles of the panopticon. Staff have to ensure that no hooks or wall hangings are present in the wards and dormitories as they could be used as ligatures by patients to hang themselves, and any suspicion of conflict between patients has to be suppressed immediately. But when there is serious overcrowding, eruptions of violence are commonplace; this was why my patient Elizabeth was so petrified at the thought of being admitted to hospital again.

Studies have been carried out to find out what patients would like in the environment of the hospital to which they have been admitted, and often, this has been a compulsory admission that their views should carry greater weight. Patients are desperate to retain their social links and need private settings for family contact and engagement. Such places should be quiet and peaceful and be clearly designated for visitors. Another important social space within the unit is a multi-faith room for religious purposes (Oeljeklaus et al., 2022).

Golembiewski (2015) describes the social aspects of a hospital setting which is patient centred and preferably patient designed. He describes this type of environment as similar to actors in a play. Staff members are, to some extent, 'backstage', not particularly prominent except in shared spaces. There are locations where staff members can be seated and observe without attracting attention so the patient is given a greater locus of control.

If you compare this with the panopticon, there are similarities. The patients are allowed space for their own purposes but are quietly observed by the staff, not in the strict way shown in the panopticon, but sensitively and without intrusion. But it all needs adequate space, and that is what is missing in most inpatient units (Babiak, 2007).

It is not always easy to find evidence that these changes in construction are beneficial in terms of outcome. Professor Tim Kendall was involved as both a planner and a clinician in developing a new locked intensive care unit (Endcliffe Ward) at one psychiatric unit in Sheffield that was formerly known to be a very disturbed and disruptive place where both staff and patients were unhappy.

So a lot of effort went into the reconstruction. The space was made much larger than the previous unit and constructed so that when any patient became acutely disturbed, they could be placed away from others without difficulty. There was ready access to the ward on foot and by a number of public transport routes, with railings to park a bicycle and a car park on-site, so that visiting as space for others to find a quiet place away from the disturbed person. There was also a 'green room' added—green has been found to be the most calming background colour, as anyone who has visited the old asylums will know. The outside area was safe and purpose built, having a leisurely appearance with secure seating and an abundance of plant life.

The consequence of this planned environmental change was that physical restraint, seclusion, and rapid tranquillisation were halved when the new unit opened, and the staff were much happier in their work there.

Disturbed patients are highly sensitive to environmental cues, and when they are placed in settings that appear homely, with (warm) coloured walls, comfortable furniture, and domestic decorations, they are more likely to be receptive to help, less suspicious, and more cooperative.

What I have described here should surprise nobody, as it only takes a modicum of thought to realise that nothing I've written is contentious; it is common sense. But we do not take any notice in most parts of the country, continue to build cramped units in inappropriate places, and then have to work out new methods of preventing the steadily increasing annual number of episodes of violence in hospitals (Khwaja & Tyrer, 2023). There is still much work to do in getting the balance right between safety requirements and the therapeutic milieu, but in addition to the general strategy of sensitively organised space, the importance of increasing natural light and display of paintings, particularly of nature, have also been found to be of benefit (Rodríguez-Labajos et al., 2024). I was made aware of the importance of paintings when caring for an Austrian patient with a wildly disinhibited personality and a recurrent psychosis. He did not like his tenth-floor flat in a high-rise building and spent very little time there, often creating disturbance in the community. But after he was left some money by a relative, he had every wall in the flat fully painted in a bright Tyrolean landscape. The effect was amazing. There was an immediate feeling of calm when you entered the flat, and everything outside seem to pale into distant insignificance. He spent much more time in the flat, was much more amenable, and often used to entertain his friends there, many of whom had mental illness and used the flat as an environmental refuge.

A similar approach has been tried with patients with such severe mental illness in Greenland that they have to be treated in Denmark. The images on many of the walls are all of icy vistas to remind them of home.

References

Arango C, Díaz-Caneja CM, McGorry PD, Rapoport J, Sommer IE, Vorstman JA, et al. (2018). Preventive strategies for mental health. *Lancet Psychiatry*, 5, 591–604.

Babiak P (2007). *Snakes in Suits: When Psychopaths Go to Work*. Harper-Collins.

Barton R (1959). *Institutional Neurosis*. John Wright.

Bentham J (1791). *Panopticon, or the Inspection House*. Bentham papers. UCL London.

Bird V, Miglietta E, Giacco D, Bauer M, Greenberg L, Lorant V, et al. (2020). Factors associated with satisfaction of inpatient psychiatric care: a cross country comparison. *Psychological Medicine*, 50, 284–292.

Deahl M (2024). General psychiatry, still in no-man's land after all these years: commentary. *British Journal of Psychiatry*, 225, 294.

Golembiewski JA (2015). Mental health facility design: the case for person-centred care. *Australian and New Zealand Journal of Psychiatry*, 49, 203–206.

Hart JT (1971). The inverse care law. *Lancet*, 297, 405–412.

Johnson S, Lamb D, Marston L, Osborn D, Mason O, Henderson C, et al. (2018). Peer-supported self-management for people discharged from a mental health crisis team: a randomised controlled trial. *Lancet*, 392, 409–418.

Khwaja M & Tyrer P (eds) (2023). *Prevention and Management of Violence: Guidance for Mental Healthcare Professionals* (2nd edition). Cambridge University Press.

Kiely B, Croke A, O'Shea M, Boland F, O'Shea E, Connolly D, et al. (2022). Effect of social prescribing link workers on health outcomes and costs for adults in primary care and community settings: a systematic review. *BMJ Open*, 12, e062951.

Marsh H (2014). *Do No Harm: Stories of Life, Death and Brain Surgery*. Weidenfeld & Nicolson.

Oeljeklaus L, Schmid HL, Kornfeld Z, Hornberg C, Norra C, Zerbe S, et al. (2022). Therapeutic landscapes and psychiatric care facilities: a qualitative meta-analysis. *International Journal of Environmental Research & Public Health*, 19, 1490.

Poole R & Huxley P (2024). Social prescribing: an inadequate response to the degradation of social care in mental health. *BJPsych Bulletin*, 48, 30–33.

Ranger M, Tyrer P, Miloseska K, Fourie H, Khaleel I, North B, et al. (2009). Cost-effectiveness of nidotherapy for comorbid personality disorder and severe mental illness: randomized controlled trial. *Epidemiologia e Psichiatria Sociale*, 18, 128–136.

Rodríguez-Labajos L, Kinloch J, Grant S, & O'Brien G (2024). The role of the built environment as a therapeutic intervention in mental health facilities: a systematic literature review. *Health Environments, Research & Design*, 17, 281–308.

Simmonds S, Coid J, Joseph P, Marriott S, & Tyrer P (2001). Community mental health team management in severe mental illness: a systematic review. *British Journal of Psychiatry*, 178, 497–502.

Thornicroft G & Tansella M (2006). Balancing community-based and hospital-based mental health care. *World Psychiatry*, 1, 84–90.

Tyrer P (1985). The hive system. A model for a psychiatric service. *British Journal of Psychiatry*, 146, 571–575.

Tyrer P (2024). *Intelligent Drug Prescribing in Psychiatry: Supporting the Patient-Prescriber Partnership*. CRC Press.

Tyrer P & Boardman J (2020). Refining social prescribing in the UK. *Lancet Psychiatry*, 7, 831–832.

Tyrer P, Crawford M, Ahmad A, Barrett B, Caan W, Duggan C, et al. (2025). A systematic environmental intervention, nidotherapy, given to whole communities: protocol for a randomised step-wedge trial. *BJPsych Open*, Apr 11;11(3):e84. doi: 10.1192/bjo.2024.861. PMID: 40214170; PMCID: PMC12052597.

Chapter 16

Adaptive approaches for Galenic syndromes

The title of this chapter may puzzle some people. What on earth are Galenic syndromes?

They are mental health problems in which personality factors, symptoms, and behaviour are so closely linked that they have to considered as single entities. Galen was a Greek physician who achieved standing in Roman society, becoming one of the foremost physicians of his age. He was really the first physician to use the scientific method when investigating disease. He joined personality to the only subjects linked to bodily function at the time, the four humours introduced by Hippocrates: black bile, yellow or red bile, blood, and phlegm. He used these as markers of illness and realised that a good diagnosis was one that predicted prognosis, 'one of the essential problems and most important objectives of Galenic diagnosis' (Mettern, 2011).

Galen was the first to understand that there was a link between the personality of an individual and bodily function. Although he was wrong, as the four humours were all wrong, he created personality types linked to each humour, and these have stuck. Too much yellow or red bile created the choleric temperament, too much black bile led to melancholia, and too much phlegm created digestive problems. Only blood, linked to good functioning and performance (hence the term 'sanguine'), was a positive humour not linked to disease.

As Galen was the first person to link personality and illness, no matter how imperfectly, he should be credited with the title of Galenic syndromes, conditions in which there is both an external component, a mental illness, and an internal component, the personality.

Importance of Galenic syndromes in practice

As studies of personality disorder in mental health services suggest that more than half of all patients assessed have personality disorders (Keown et al., 2002), even though this may not be recognised as these are seldom diagnosed, it is likely that Galenic syndromes could occur by chance. But

DOI: 10.4324/9781003560630-16

there are some conditions in which the elements of personality and mental disorders are so closely linked that they cannot usefully be separated. A true Galenic syndrome is 'a combination of personality disorder and clinical symptom complex so frequently associated that the two conditions should be considered as a single disorder' (Tyrer et al., 2022).

This concept is new, but here are three common Galenic syndromes with their descriptions, followed by case examples showing how they are managed with nidotherapy.

The general neurotic syndrome

This term is not commonly known but it defines accurately the common presentation of unpleasant symptoms, mainly anxiety and depression, and personality problems in the negative affective and anankastic domains. I described it first in a paper published in the *Lancet* in 1985:

> [I]t is more appropriate to regard many of these conditions (i.e., neuroses) as manifestations of one disorder, which may be termed the 'general neurotic syndrome'. To qualify for this diagnosis patients should show at least three of the following features:
>
> (a) two or more of the following symptomatic diagnoses are present together, either now or at times in the past: agoraphobia and social phobias, panic disorder, non-psychotic depression, anxiety, and hypochondriasis (including somatoform disorders);
> (b) at least one episode of illness has developed in the absence of major stress;
> (c) There are abnormal personality features of a passive dependent or an anankastic type;
> (d) There is a history of a similar syndrome in first-degree relatives.
>
> (Tyrer, 1985)

The definition I gave was too precise; the general neurotic syndrome is better summarised as anxiety, depression and, neuroticism. This is a standard Galenic syndrome with a very close combination of mental symptoms with personality domains. Readers who want to know more about the science that underpins it can read about it elsewhere (Tyrer, 2022). But it is well illustrated by Vivienne, who was first seen by me at the beginning of the Nottingham Study of Neurotic Disorder in 1983 when she was 21. At that time, she was very distressed after marital separation and a series of unsatisfactory jobs where she had been bullied. Full assessment showed that she was both anxious and depressed with periods of panic and great uncertainty about her future.

Assessment of her personality showed she had a strong tendency to rely on others for support, even though they very frequently let her down, and she had been persistently anxious since the age of eight. Her mother was also chronically anxious.

She did not make much progress over the following two years and had periods when she felt totally alone and was suicidal. I had not grasped the principles of nidotherapy at that time and was stuck about finding any solution, but I could see that in the absence of stable relationships, her life would be likely to continue in the same mode. When she asked me what might help, in one of my musings, I suggested glibly and without much thought, 'You need to meet a good man'.

Some five years after this, she went through more distress after a relationship with a man who was certainly not good to her or for her, whom she had left after he became abusive. She became agoraphobic and was admitted to a general hospital after an overdose of antidepressants and was looked after by a male nurse later after being admitted to a psychiatric ward. She was surprised by how much sympathy he showed her, but within a week, she was discharged. Nearly two years later, Vivienne took another overdose and was admitted to the same hospital.

Quite by chance, she was later admitted to the same psychiatric ward and looked after by the same male nurse. He recognised her immediately, and during this admission, she explained, or rather off-loaded, all her problems to him. She was certain this would put him off her entirely, but he asked to continue seeing her after she left hospital. They fell in love and were married shortly afterward. Her life completely changed at that point. She had a secure relationship with a loving partner and lost almost all her symptoms. Unfortunately, despite several years of a happy marriage, he became ill and died 3 years before Vivienne was seen at the 30-year follow-up point of our research study. She had a return of some of her symptoms but not to the same extent as when first seen.

Without going into too much detail. it is easy to see why this account combines personality and symptoms so intimately. It is impossible to separate Vivienne's personality from her symptoms of anxiety, depression, and panic and similarly difficult to ignore her symptoms in describing her personality.

The Aristippean syndrome

The Aristippean syndrome combines the personality domains of impulsiveness and dissociality with substance misuse. It is present in a minor form in the case of Callum, described in Chapter 1. Here is a second case example.

John was also involved in the Nottingham Study of Neurotic Disorder. His personality status at entry was rated as severe personality disorder, and when I saw him, I could only sympathise with a man who had derived nothing but conflict from his life. He was chronically angry, anxious, and depressed; was taking large doses of benzodiazepines and antidepressants with very little effect apart from temporary highs; and was suffused with hate about the way he had been treated by his parents, who had always favoured his younger brother. This anger extended to all members of the family. He continued to be unwell up to the 12-year follow up point, and it looked as though he would have a very poor outcome at 30 years.

He then experienced what could be described as an epiphany moment. At a time when he was feeling more depressed than he had ever done, he took it on himself to walk into a Catholic Church in Nottingham. He sat down in one of the pews, and a priest came to see him. John professed to no religious faith but found the presence of the priest comforting, and when he left, he was given a rosary. He left the church and, quite suddenly, made the decision to change his life around. He was going to forget all the past troubles at home and forge a new life for himself. He also resolved to stop all his medication and start afresh with no pharmacological help.

It was a great struggle to get off all his medication, taking nearly 2 years, but he succeeded. He joined an allotment group, made new friends there who knew nothing about his past, and became highly competent at gardening. At the 30-year follow-up, he could not properly explain what had happened—only that seeing the priest had given him the realisation that he could have a different life. When he was assessed, he had symptom scores all below the threshold of pathology and had good social function.

The Diogenes or Greta Garbo syndrome

'I want to be alone' is the most famous statement of Greta Garbo. Although it was made in a film, it also reflected her opinion when fame overwhelmed her. The Diogenes syndrome is sometimes attached to a condition called hoarding disorder, but as you will gather from reading Chapter 7, this is completely inappropriate, and Greta Garbo should more properly be attached to this syndrome of detachment and major pathology, in whom the subject, in the DSM system, would be regarded as schizotypal.

Case example of the Greta Garbo Galenic syndrome

Anthea was first seen by me in 1988 when I joined a new community service in London, which visited almost all its patients at home in the first instance. It took some time to get access to her flat as we had been warned that she was difficult to engage.

Eventually, after several failed attempts, a slight, shadowy, slim figure could be seen coming to the front door. It was Anthea. She was fearful.

'Are you here to take me into hospital?' she said in a resigned voice. 'No, Anthea', we replied; we are from the early intervention service, and our task is to keep people out of hospital'. This was a good start and enough for her to let us into the flat.

Once we were inside her flat, we had a pleasant surprise. It was a very comfortable home: neat carpets, elegant bookcases filled with the works of well-known writers, a small but well-stocked kitchen, and comfortable chairs. Anthea was a cultured and amusing individual with an interesting view on life—she regarded the world as an enemy with which she was in combat—and, despite clearly being isolated, was very proud to show off her flat to these unexpected visitors. She had an impressive variety of fish in her aquarium, had a piano that she played beautifully, had elegant book-cases filled with the works of erudite writers, and attended evening even-song at St Paul's cathedral every Sunday. She was fluent in four languages and had a fund of experiences to tell us about life in Somerset, where she had previously been treated.

But this was where the sad story started. She was brought up in Som-erset and had a much older brother. Her detached personality developed early; she had few friends at school and was only interested in art and literature, spending long periods walking in the countryside. Her life was rather like that of Emily Brontë, the sister in the Brontë family who was always considered strange and a bit of an outcast, and it was only when she obtained a university place in Amsterdam that she felt her life could start properly.

Unfortunately, at the age of 21, while in Amsterdam, she developed her first psychotic episode, a mixture of wild over-activity, auditory hallucina-tions of strange interlopers inside her head, and devilish beliefs. She was admitted to hospital and transferred back to Somerset and, for the next 17 years, had a compulsory admission to hospital for at least a short time every year. Each of these admissions was preceded by an acute psychotic episode, followed by a period in hospital when she was sedated, was given antipsychotic drugs, and improved but then preferred to be mute as she was afraid anything she said would lead to more medication being prescribed. All this history was backed up by the previous records from the Somerset Hos-pital. Once out of hospital, she was said to be 'persistently non-compliant with treatment' and never kept any outpatient appointments.

Anthea told us that she never took a single tablet of medication once she had been discharged as she regarded all the treatment as a form of poison; it 'completely upset my hormones'. She had a brief marriage in her late 20s and, largely because of her repeated illness episodes, had been divorced by her husband. She had a son, and although she tried hard to care for him, the impact of her repeated admissions and lack of other carers led to him being taken into care by social services.

We further explored her continued refusal to keep any appointments as an outpatient, despite invariably agreeing to keep appointments before she left hospital. She knew from all the conversations she had with doctors about her problem that antipsychotic drug treatment would always be recommended because she had a disorder within the schizophrenia spectrum. She felt the only way she could ever leave hospital was to passively agree with all the medical advice offered, even though she had no intention of complying with the instructions once she had left hospital. Our assessment, established without too much difficulty, was that she had a disorder within the schizophrenia spectrum and also a detached personality that was moderately but not grossly severe.

At this point, the average clinician would almost certainly abandon Anthea as another example of the frustrations created by patients refusing sound advice, quietly retire from the scene, and wait for the next psychotic episode.

But we had more time than most at our service to reflect on the management of patients like Anthea. We continued to see her at her flat and felt that, with strong advocacy, we could at least persuade her to take antipsychotic drugs, if only as required, as soon as there was the slightest evidence of a return of her illness. In giving this advice, we were following a good evidence base; acute psychosis is very difficult to treat in any other way.

Anthea listened patiently but would not budge. If she was going to have to be admitted to hospital every year, that was fate at work; she would not try to avoid it by taking poisonous drugs. This was the point at which nidotherapy was born. The physical and social environment that Anthea had been living in for most of her life was a toxic one of a series of upheavals in which she had virtually no control. The fact that she could be regarded as partly to blame for this by refusing to take preventive medication was unimportant; she had strong reasons for refusing, and we had to listen to them.

So we went into detail about her past experiences, assessing not only her personality function but also the pattern of her illness. What was clear from this analysis was that the actual duration of her psychotic episodes was likely to be very short, probably no more than a few days. Although most of her hospital admissions lasted about three months, it seemed likely this length of time was unnecessary. Anthea appeared to get better very quickly if her testimony was to be believed, but because she made the mistake of mute passive cooperation when in hospital, the clinical staff probably presumed she was still ill and continued her detention accordingly.

In addition to these episodes being very brief, they were followed by a full recovery. This was unusual. When patients with schizophrenia have had many admissions to hospital, they usually have some degree of what are called negative symptoms, labelled negative as they include loss of drive, apathy, lack if pleasure in any activity, and slow, monotonous speech with little variation. But Anthea's behaviour was the antithesis of this. She was lively, polylingual, socially aware despite having no real friends, and a good companion.

This led to the conclusion that this was not typical schizophrenia and also allowed us to recommend a completely new treatment plan. We introduced a 'hunker-down strategy' for her episodes of illness, asking her to ensure she had enough provisions in her house so she could lock herself at home whenever she became unwell. As she had a short premonitory period before each episode, she was able to anticipate it to some extent. Once she was in the middle of her psychotic episodes, she was advised not to leave her house as it would be likely that her behaviour would lead to alarm and possible compulsory detention.

As an additional measure, I also wrote a letter for her to have available at all times and to bring it with here whenever she happened to be admitted to hospital in the future.

This included the lines 'Anthea has a tendency to experience very brief psychotic episodes that only last a few days. Could you please note this if she is admitted to hospital as she can probably be discharged very quickly. She refuses antipsychotic medication when well'.

This worked well. The next 28 years of Anthea's life were dramatically changed from the previous 28. She changed her name to Avis to mark the advent of a new persona. Her detached personality remained, but as her confidence improved, she developed a new friend. At one event, she came across 'a pink lady' and asked me to get in contact with her afterwards a she was sure they would get on well. The pink lady, who always preferred pink in all her clothes, certainly acted as an attractive beacon for Anthea/Avis, and on one occasion, I was invited with Anthea/Avis to a marvellous dinner in Earl's Court. Anthea/Avis continued to have brief episodes of psychosis but was never in hospital for more than a few days. A correspondent who wrote 'I would not like to be in Professor Tyrer's shoes when his psychotic patient on no drugs is violent and relapses' need not have worried.

We also established contact with her son, an undergraduate at Cambridge University, and they were reunited; she became an excellent mosaic artist, had her works exhibited with one bought by the actor Ricky Gervais, and also took part in a number of not very good plays written by me and performed in London. I had a meeting with Jonathan Miller, the famous director, and he told me the plays were 'not bad, but the actors were awful'. I had to admit to him that the plays were written for the patients as part of an approach called nidotherapy and the quality was less important than the pleasure of performance.

Anthea died eight years ago from multiple myeloma, her last (pre-terminal) episode of psychosis while an inpatient alarming the staff at the National Hospital for Nervous Diseases as it was so unexpected, but, as we already knew, it only lasted a few days. (In this account, I have not disguised any information as Anthea gave me full permission to write about her experiences many years before she died. 'I want others to know more about me and how it is possible to fight the system', she told me. When I responded, 'If you had listened to the tiny part of the system that asked you to take a small dose of medication as soon as you became ill, you would have saved yourself a lot of trouble', she retorted, 'If I did that, you would never have known what I was really like'.)

This long account of a Galenic syndrome might lead some psychiatrists to comment, 'Who does Tyrer think we are? We have to see dozens of patients every day and whether they have personality problems or not has very little meaning for us. We have to deal with what is put in front of us. We do not have the luxury of time that allows us to look at every nook and cranny of a patient's past. It is just unreasonable to expect this from us'.

But I argue that if you want to be stimulated in your profession and excited by the novelty of differences, then addressing both the personalities and the clinical syndromes of patients gives you the extra facet that converts a two-dimensional assessment into a three-dimensional one.

The other advantage of knowing something more about the personalities of the patients who are sometimes difficult to treat is that you are much more likely to work in harness with them in a collaborative manner than if you just concentrate on treating the overt mental illness. In all the examples I have discussed, "that recognizing mental illness alone was insufficient for choosing the best treatment" Understanding the personalities behind the illness was an important asset in finding a solution.

References

Keown P, Holloway F, & Kuipers E (2002). The prevalence of personality disorders, psychotic disorders and affective disorders amongst the patients seen by a community mental health team in London. *Social Psychiatry and Psychiatric Epidemiology*, 37, 225–229.

Mettern S (2011). Galen and his patients. *Lancet*, 378, 478–479.

Tyrer P (1985). Neurosis divisible? *Lancet*, 325, 685–688.

Tyrer P (2022). *Neurosis: Understanding Common Mental Illness*. Cambridge University Press.

Tyrer P, Mulder R, Newton-Howes G, & Duggan C (2022). Galenic syndromes: combinations of mental state and personality disorders too closely entwined to be separated. *British Journal of Psychiatry*, 220, 309–310.

Chapter 17

Adapting to unstable environments

In Chapter 1, I described how species of plants achieve success by adapting to different environments in ways that promote their numbers. If the environments are temporary, unstable ones, their success may be short lived as the adaptation will no longer fit. This phenomenon in the plant kingdom is described as plant succession. Let us take one common example of this phenomenon.

There is a very attractive common marsh and wet grassland plant called meadowsweet. It is bright cream with white flowers and neat, aromatic leaves and thrives in places where its roots are constantly underwater. But over time, the climate may change, or the decaying roots may raise the soil level so it is no longer marshy, and then plants more suited to dry conditions will take over. The environment in the end holds the answers, showing that adaptation is never completely fixed. There are always dynamic changes, and these apply to personal and social aspects of the environment as well as physical ones.

Here are some common environmental changes that require adjustive adaptation.

1. Sudden career success

In the media, this is most obviously seen with celebrity culture. Celebrities are the brittle reminders of the consequences of instant fame, shown most often with pop music idols, sports stars, charismatic politicians, and film stars. When you are suddenly raised to the top of the tree, there are only two options: you work very hard to stay among the high branches without slipping, or you fall to a lower level.

Staying up is difficult, and when it is successful, it needs a new form of adaptation to keep it there. Often adaptation fails. In 2006, David Owen (the same David Owen who used to be a junior doctor working for the same consultant as I did) described the hubris syndrome and later (Owen & Davidson, 2009; Owen, 2012) defined it as an acquired personality disorder

DOI: 10.4324/9781003560630-17

and listed its characteristics, hoping its operational criteria might find their way into a new edition of the *Diagnostic and Statistical Manual for Mental Disorders* (Table 18.1). He was very generous in allocating attribution to this disorder, and in keeping with his position as a former minister in government, he assessed his fellow politicians. David Owen's conclusion was that in the UK, Herbert Asquith, David Lloyd George, Neville Chamberlain, Winston Churchill, Anthony Eden, Margaret Thatcher, and Tony

Table 18.1 A comparison of the characteristics of the hubris syndrome in politicians and celebrities of instant fame

Politicians (after Owen, 2012)	Celebrities
1. A narcissistic propensity to see the world as an arena in which to exercise power and seek glory	1. A narcissistic propensity to see the world as a stage for their own advancement
2. A predisposition to take actions which seem likely to cast the individual in a good light	2. An advertising machine that promotes the individual in a good light
3. A disproportionate concern with image and presentation	3. Excessive attention to self-publicity
4. A messianic manner of talking about current activities and a tendency to exaltation	4. Promotional activities that go far beyond the substance of their success
5. Identification with the organisation to the extent that the individual regards his/her outlook and interests as identical	5. Promotion of a following that slavishly tracks progress of the celebrity and promotes cult-like worship
6. A tendency to speak in the third person or use the royal 'we'	6. The celebrity becomes an independent entity
7. Excessive confidence in the individual's own judgment and contempt for the advice or criticism of others	7. Over-confidence in the ability to replicate the initial achievements that first led to fame
8. Exaggerated self-belief, bordering on a sense of omnipotence	8. Exaggerated self-belief that lacks justification but is reinforced by others
9. An unshakable belief that, in the court of public opinion, they will be vindicated	9. The belief that the support of their fans will overcome all obstacles
10. Loss of contact with reality often associated with progressive isolation	10. The isolation that comes with fame leads to over-reaching ambition
11. Restlessness, recklessness, and impulsiveness	11. Rash adventures after poor advice
12. A tendency to allow their 'broad vision' about the moral rectitude of a proposed course to obviate the need to consider practicality, cost, or outcomes	12. Extension of interest beyond the limits of their innate abilities to areas where they are ignorant

Blair all had the disorder, and in the US, Theodore Roosevelt, Woodrow Wilson, Franklin D. Roosevelt, John F. Kennedy. Lyndon B Johnson, Richard Nixon, and George W. Bush all had the same syndrome too. David Owen selected his acquired personality types before Donald Trump came on the scene. How unfortunate. Examination of Table 18.1 shows that Donald would live up to his name by trumping all the others in the list to become the unchallenged hubris leader ('After all, I am your favourite president').

David Owen hit on something important, and I can understand his reasons for labelling it as an acquired personality disorder, one that he surmised would disappear when the environment changed. But this overstates the argument. What happens frequently when people are suddenly thrust into the spotlight of fame is a failure to adjust to the new environment. The hubris syndrome is negative nidotherapy, an environmental change that upsets the equilibrium of the personality and leads to a temporary maladjustment, and it can be found in many who desperately wish for their names to be on everybody's lips and then cannot adjust to the consequences when they happen.

The characteristics are not just confined to politicians (Table 18.1). There is no need for me to give examples of people who are thrust into the limelight of instant success and shortly afterwards plummet into despond, often to early death. They are littered across the news. Adapting to sudden change, whether it is positive or negative, throws a wrench in to your repertoire of adjustment that is not easy to accommodate. Having someone close to you who is not in the limelight, who can advise and support without the need for empty worship, such as Rosalynn Carter was to her husband, Jimmy, both when he was US President and afterward, is an invaluable asset.

But the need to be aware of environmental change is not just confined to figures of importance. It applies to everybody. 'Be careful what you wish for', runs the cautionary phrase, 'it may happen and spoil the show'. There are many examples of those with personality difficulties adapting well to temporary changes after becoming successful, only to be dashed by failure when the environment changes, and personality adaptation cannot keep up. In the Nottingham study of neurotic disorder, we came across many examples of apparently stable environment changing in ways that turned out to be pathological in the long term and led to problems in adjustment. Here is one example that could have been repeated many times.

Jane lived in a council house in the centre of Nottingham. She suffered from intermittent anxiety and depression in the early years of the follow-up study when she was very timid and felt undervalued and was also subservient to her husband. She put a lot of her symptoms down to her poor marital relationship, but part of it related to her tendency to be over dependent. Jeff, her husband, spent most of his spare time drinking with friends and was frequently abusive and casually violent. Jane tolerated this while her children were young but filed for divorce when her husband found another partner. For the first time in her life, she felt better and adapted the council house to suit her needs, found a part-time job, and most of her depressive and anxiety symptoms resolved. Her children remained at home, and, partly because they were very comfortable there and because of local housing difficulties, two of them continue to stay at home when grown-up and working.

When one of them was married, he asked to stay with his wife at Jane's home; she felt she could not refuse. But her neat and well-ordered house now seemed to be changing into a cramped and crammed lodging place and no longer had its former attraction; the meadowsweet was being invaded by thistles. So Jane asked Nottingham council if she could be rehoused.

Although this was desired, when it came, the outcome was disappointing. She was moved to a new housing estate five miles from the centre of Nottingham that was poorly served by public transport. Her children continue to live their own lives and rarely visited. She became more isolated and alone than she had ever been before. At the 30-year follow-up point in the Nottingham study, she did not answer the door despite many knocks and rings. It was only after checking with neighbours that we returned to try again. 'Why didn't you answer the door earlier?' She explained, 'I've given up answering; nobody ever calls'. This follow-up took place five years after she had moved.

It is not difficult to see how Jane's natural dependence led to problems initially after her marriage and also to those she experienced after she moved to her new address, with only the middle years satisfying her needs to be dependent but also closely involved with her children. You may rightly say that it cannot be the task of a nidotherapist to anticipate all these changes in the environment when offering advice. But if Jane had been exposed to adaptive discussions in the knowledge of her personality structure, some of these difficulties might have been avoided. It is possible to argue it was unwise for her to change accommodation without a better appreciation of the options available and the recognition of her need for support and reinforcement. It is equally possible to say that the changes she went through were the slings and arrows of outrageous fortune that we all have to experience and come to terms in our own way. But, rather like steering a boat in a choppy sea, if you have developed skills in counteracting these environmental waves and adjusting to them, you have more control and are in the better position to preserve your autonomy.

Sudden adversity

There are as many environments of adversity as those of success, if not more. They can occur in the physical environment—earthquakes, floods, fire, and storms—the social environment—loss of employment, broken relationships, death or serious illness of a loved one—and the personal environment—humiliation, persecution, and dishonour.

Adaptation to dramatically changed circumstances will need people to draw on all their personality strengths, particularly those of determination, emotional strengths, and discernment, that allow them to see beyond immediate hardships and privations and find compensatory adjustments. Because there are so many different ways in which adversity may be shown, it is not possible to give adaptation strategies except in the broadest sense.

In addressing their needs, the person has to determine if the adverse events are temporary or permanent. If they are temporary, there is no reason existing adaptation procedures should not continue; soldiering on to the end is perfectly appropriate, and any deflections from existing plans need only be temporary.

There is also abundant evidence that help from others is much more likely at times of acute privation and stress (Judt, 2010) and has also been shown in laboratory studies (von Dawans et al., 2012). The consequences include improved social cohesion, so if the adversity becomes a shared one, support is also shared and reinforcing.

There are also some highly negative environments in which people can become enmeshed and from which they find it difficult to escape. Help may be needed in these.

The Peter Principle, named after Laurence Peter, a Canadian economist, states that '(M)embers of a hierarchy are promoted until they reach the level at which they are no longer competent' (Peter & Hull, 1969). This can sometimes include those who are promoted until they reach a level when they think they are no longer competent (even though they are). This second group has been defined as the impostor (or imposter) syndrome.

The hierarchy of occupational systems, particularly large ones, can be like prisons from which it is very difficult to escape.

Here is an example.

Bruce was a successful and popular boy at school, excelling in several sports and working hard at his studies, which he found trying at times. His parents wanted him to be a doctor and gave him strong encouragement to pursue a medical career. As he was a worrier, he was attracted to a specialty where he would be financially secure. But underneath, he always wanted to be outside in the open air with less pressure to study, and he had the fantasy of becoming an explorer and an adventurer. But, with pressure from both the school and his parents, he studied medicine at university and became a doctor. He became dependent on others' good wishes and advice and, without really having any long-term plans, was persuaded to apply and become a clinical lecturer at a medical school, where he specialised in virology.

He was good at teaching, but he was also expected to carry out research and provide income for the university. His wife, who was a fellow academic in social sciences, pushed him to study more and involved him in some of her work, where she was beginning to excel. He complied with these pressures and had some success, so he was promoted to senior lecturer. But this only increased the pressure to do more, and he became depressed and increasingly anxious, particularly when presenting his research data to colleagues, as he thought it was poor and lacking any merit.

He had difficulty sleeping, his concentration suffered, and his depression became so intense at time he was suicidal. Then, almost out of the blue, he was invited to Romania to help in resolving an outbreak of West Nile viral infection, a disease transmitted by birds but which can infect humans and lead to serious neurological problems. He stayed with a family at the edge of a forest in Transylvania. He was in his element in this environment and was completely invigorated. The West Nile infection was resolved, but he stayed on to help with the reforestation of the region and decided to give up his medical career. He fell in love with the daughter of his mentor in Transylvania and made the difficult decision to leave his wife and remarry. His life had completely changed, and the general neurotic syndrome that had dogged him all his life had disappeared.

There are others in some walks of life who always have ups and downs in their lives. Politicians are an example. Enoch Powell said that every politician's life ends in failure, and he is almost always right. Benjamin Disraeli likened his advancement to prime minister to being on top of the greasy pole—it is very easy to slide down again into oblivion.

It is too early to conclude that the current environment in which Donald Trump thrives is a temporary one, but many people across the world will be watching closely. But, taking a more distant perspective, it seems highly unlikely that a person who castigates and bullies others to get his own way, who lies to prevent the admission of failure, who takes more notice of his gut feelings than of the expertise of others, and who rules by chaos and division will continue to survive in a different environment. So when this environment changes, as indeed is very likely at some point, the Trumpian qualities of attack, blame, and threaten will no longer be effective. As there is no nidotherapist on earth who could deflect Donald Trump' powerful personality characteristics into more collaborative activities, it looks as though a major environmental change is going to be needed to change direction.

References

Judt T (2010). *The Memory Chalet*. New York: The Penguin Press.

Owen D (2012). *The Hubris Syndrome: Bush, Blair and the Intoxication of Power*. Methuen.

Owen D & Davidson J (2009). Hubris syndrome: an acquired personality disorder? a study of US Presidents and UK Prime Ministers over the last 100 years. *Brain*, 132, 1396–1406.

Peter LJ & Hull R (1969). *The Peter Principle*. Pan Books.

von Dawans B, Fischbacher U, Kirschbaum C, Fehr E, & Heinrichs M (2012). The social dimension of stress reactivity: acute stress increases prosocial behavior in humans. *Psychological Science*, 23, 651–660.

Chapter 18

The treatment of severe personality disorder

I have left this chapter to the end because it is the most difficult subject in the book.

This is the bald description of severe personality disorder from the ICD-11 revision of the classification of personality disorders:

All general diagnostic requirements for personality disorder are met.

- There are severe disturbances in multiple areas of functioning of the self (e.g. sense of self may be so unstable that individuals report not having a sense of who they are, or so rigid that they refuse to participate in any but an extremely narrow range of situations; self-view may be characterised by self-contempt or be grandiose or highly eccentric; see Box 6.2).
- Problems in interpersonal functioning seriously affect virtually all relationships, and the ability and willingness to perform expected social and occupational roles is severely compromised or absent.
- Specific manifestations of personality disturbance affect most, if not all, areas of personality functioning.
- Severe personality disorder is often associated with harm to self or others.
- Severe personality disorder is associated with severe impairment in all or nearly all areas of life, including personal, family, social, educational, occupational and other important areas of functioning.

There is also an additional section:

Examples of specific personality disturbances in severe personality disorder

The individual's self-view is very unrealistic and is typically highly unstable or contradictory.

DOI: 10.4324/9781003560630-18

The individual has serious difficulty with regulation of self-esteem, emotional experience and expression, and impulses, as well as other aspects of behaviour (e.g. perseveration, indecision).

The individual is largely unable to set and pursue realistic goals.

The individual's interpersonal relationships, if any, lack mutuality; they are shallow, extremely one-sided, unstable or highly conflictual, often to the point of violence. Family relationships are absent (despite having living relatives) or marred by significant conflict.

The individual has extreme difficulty acknowledging difficult or unwanted emotions (e.g. does not recognise or acknowledge experiencing anger, sadness or other emotions).

The individual is unwilling or unable to sustain regular work due to lack of interest or effort, poor performance (e.g. failure to complete assignments or perform expected roles, unreliability), interpersonal difficulties or inappropriate behaviour (e.g. fits of temper, insubordination).

Under stress, there are extreme distortions in the individual's situational and interpersonal appraisals. There are often dissociative states or psychotic-like beliefs or perceptions (e.g. extreme paranoid reactions).

(World Health Organisation, 2024, p. 558)

This combination is quite a toxic bundle, and it is not yet known how many in the population would qualify for this diagnosis. Preliminary evidence shows it is rare. It is also worth emphasising that people can still qualify for the diagnosis by only having a certain proportion of the characteristics listed here. The only two epidemiological studies that have reported this in general populations give figures of 1.3% (Yang et al., 2010) and 0.9% (Bach et al., 2023). Most people with severe personality disorders had very disturbed and often traumatic childhoods. In the first of these studies, of the 109 people identified with severe personality disorder (from a UK population of nearly 9,000 chosen at random), every single one of these 109 had conduct disorder as children, a condition often found in disturbed families in which there is serious antisocial and aggressive behaviour leading to major disruption.

If one in a hundred people has severe personality problems, you may think you should see them fairly frequently. This is not so. One of the populations that has a high proportion is the homeless. In one review, between 64% and 79% were judged to have a personality disorder (Neves Horácio et al., 2023), but as severity was not recorded, the proportions with this level of disorder is not known. Most of those with such severe disorders have very little contact with other people. If you have serious disruption in every aspect of your life, there is unlikely to be meaningful interaction with other people; you become an outcast.

But it is still possible for those with severe personality disorder to adapt and succeed. I will give you two examples: one historical, which involved the person acting as his own nidotherapist, the second, very different, a current problem needing much extra help.

Example 1. Ludwig van Beethoven

Ludwig was born in Bonn, Germany, in 1770. His father, Johann van Beethoven, came from Flanders in Belgium. He was a fairly talented musician and singer, played the violin and zither, and taught music at court. But he was also a heavy drinker, developed alcohol dependence, became bad tempered, and was not much involved with his seven children. The Beethoven family home was not a happy one, but Johann was perceptive enough to recognise that his son, Ludwig, was a gifted musician and promoted him as much as possible, made him practise constantly on the piano, and tried to portray him as another child genius like Wolfgang Amadeus Mozart. Ludwig's musical training began when he was four. The regime was harsh and intensive, with irregular late-night sessions with the young Beethoven dragged from his bed half asleep to practise on the keyboard. It was reported on one occasion, standing on a stool to reach the keys, he was beaten for every missed note, a repeated torture that went on throughout the night.

Johann got into financial difficulty and attempted to defraud the heirs of the first minister of the court by forging the signature of the minister and was exposed but not convicted.

Ludwig had to take over the running of the family and once had to intervene with the police to prevent his father being taken into custody.

So poor Ludwig had a bad start in life. But his music saved him, even though the scars of the past could not be erased. He gained a reputation as a virtuoso pianist and moved to Vienna. Although he was soon patronised by the nobility of the city and composed for them, he became disenchanted with the shallowness of his work. By now he had developed all the characteristics of a complex personality disorder. He, like his father and grandfather before him, drank alcohol to excess, became irritable and angry, and fell out with his patrons. But he retained a high opinion of himself, and this kept him going. In one well-known riposte he said his patron, Prince Karl von Lichnowsky, 'Prince, what you are you are by accident of birth; what I am I am through myself. There have been and still will be thousands of princes; there is only one Beethoven'.

He never married. His famous piece *Für Elise* was not found until 40 years after his death and was probably written for a young woman he had hoped to marry, but there was little evidence that the relationship ever developed into a close one. For much of his life, he was isolated and detached and had no close friends. He was also markedly impulsive. When he decided that his artistic freedom was being compromised by having to compose pieces for his patrons that did not inspire, he suddenly decided to become an independent musician, probably the first at the time in the world. At this point in his life, he was beginning to show signs of his later deafness, but he still threw away the shackles of patronage and composed as he wished. It worked, and he soon returned to financial security.

Beethoven was also incredibly meticulous and obsessional. He wrote and rewrote many of his scores dozens of times before settling on a final one. His obsessionality also influenced his personal life. This showed itself in particular in his washing rituals. At these times, he would sing at the top of his voice and pour buckets of water over his head. As this was not carried out over a sink or any other receptacle, the water used to leak through the floor and cause consternation to the people below.

It seems likely that Beethoven had pathological degrees of all the five personality domains described in this book. It is uncertain whether he would be described as having severe personality disorder as his musical talent allowed him good contact with his peers and a sufficient income. But when we hear about his personal circumstances, they are very like those who have lost contact with normal society.

He rarely stayed in any one house for long. He had no interest in warmth, good food, or other domestic comforts, and he lived in a state of complete disorder. He ceased to pay any attention to his clothes, on one occasion coming to give a musical lesson to a young woman in a dressing gown, slippers, and a peaked nightcap, and those who knew him well used to smuggle clothes into his wardrobe, knowing he would hardly recognise them and wear them the following day.

In an film broadcast on Sky Arts, *Beethoven and Me*, which was named best music programme in the 2022 Broadcast Awards, I was interviewed by Charles Hazlewood, the well-known conductor of the Paraorchestra. Charles felt a strong affinity with Beethoven as he too was abused as a child. In his interview with me, we concluded that Ludwig van Beethoven, for most of his life, had a moderately severe personality disorder with the domains of negative affectivity, detachment, and anankastia being particularly prominent. As personality disorder is capable of shifting over time, I think it highly likely in his later years that he probably had severe personality disorder.

But, according to the diagnostic requirements, this would mean that he had 'severe impairment in all or nearly all areas of life, including personal, family, social, educational, occupational and other important areas of functioning'. Yes, but 'nearly all' is the key couplet. His personal, family, and social lives were an utter mess, but he was still able to work, and his personality problems may well have turned out to be assets at this time. I commented earlier on the value of personality strengths; Beethoven had the strengths of determination, independence, and discernment in abundance. He knew where he wanted to go and was going to remove the obstacles that were placed in his way, and no one was going to stop him.

Beethoven had never heard of nidotherapy, but he was practising it for most of his adult life. He encountered lots of obstacles, removed or got round most of them, and emerged triumphant on the other side. He adapted the environment to accommodate his personality and his talent, and the world was a much better place as a consequence.

Example 2. Melanie Lukeman

Melanie is 47. She is not seeking fame and does not feel she has abundant talent, but she is as determined as Beethoven in her own way. At present, her nidotherapy management and her adaptive abilities are still being tested, but in addressing them, we can get a better understanding of severe personality problems and how they are appreciated in different settings.

Her childhood, like those of so many with severe personality disorder, was a deprived and brutal one. She has never known her father, who disappeared from her life very soon after her birth. Her mother was a barmaid who had many casual sexual relationships and had three children with different partners, of whom Melanie was one. At the age of three, Melanie suffered her first sexual abuse with a lorry driver, a person her mother had approved to look after Melanie. There were frequent drunken fights at their home, and Melanie has repeated early images of stabbings and blood all over the kitchen floor. When she was five, she found a cupboard at home where she could hide and escape the furor outside, and this became her safe haven over many years that followed.

Later, she was befriended by another man who asked her to touch herself down below and recorded all her movements with a camera. Later, he used video recordings and gave her presents for her help with his filming. She had no idea of his motives and just followed his instructions blindly. Because her mother gave the family so little attention, Melanie was asked to look after her brothers and sisters for much of the time, a task which helped stabilise her.

There were frequent beatings in the house with another of her mother's lovers, and Melanie learnt to hide her younger brother in the cupboard as he was so disturbed by the screams. The man concerned was subsequently charged with rape and was committed to Broadmoor Hospital. Her mother used to visit him there, and Melanie served as a drug mule for him when visiting with her mother.

Her mother was later admitted to hospital, and Melanie and her brothers and sisters were fostered on three occasions. On one of these occasions the foster parents were very kind, and Melanie pleaded to be able to stay with them as this was the first time she had ever received proper love and affection. But because her mother later came out of hospital, she had to return home.

She received inconsistent schooling and, after being fostered again at the age of 15, was not able to complete her education. Despite this, she did not do badly at school and received an A-plus GCSE in physical education. She ran away from home at the age of 16 and shortly afterwards became pregnant; she subsequently had other brief relationships and had three children. Unfortunately none of these turned out well, and she remined single. Her son Cory died at the age of three from meningitis. She has had two sons since, Leo and Reece; Reece has been a key nidotherapist in her care.

Melanie's mental health problems could be said to have begun at the age of 6, but she first presented to psychiatric services at the age of 18. She was diagnosed as having emotionally unstable personality disorder, and although she responded to a course of cognitive behaviour therapy between 2005 and 2008, she subsequently relapsed, and her emotional instability led to a series of self-harming events.

This became a serious behavioural pattern in 2022. Early in the year, she took an overdose of medication and had to be admitted to an intensive care unit when she was placed in of the Mental Health Act. The trust were concerned about her care but were reluctant to allocate her a care coordinator even though she qualified for the enhanced care programme approach. After further consultation and as a response to what was called a 'procedural lacuna', there were further discussions.

Then, in a curious circumlocutory argument, the trust, at a joint meeting, argued the case that a care coordinator was not necessary:

> M is not currently eligible for the CPA as her needs are being managed with a clear treatment plan. In any event, allocating a care coordinator would not offer any clinical benefit to M and in fact would potentially be detrimental to her; given her condition of emotionally unstable personality disorder and dependent personality traits a care coordinator would feed existing attachment and dependency issues and there would also be a risk of destabilisation if the care coordinator were to move to another role. As such, the Trust would be failing in its duty of care to M if it were to allocate her a care coordinator.

Stage 1 in nidotherapy—establishing the relationship

Because the trust had, in effect, abandoned care for Melanie, our charity, NIDUS-UK, decided to take on her care—mainly in the form of my input. I realised this was not going to be an easy task, and it only was agreed after I had a four-hour assessment of Melanie at a local community centre. This represented the first phase of nidotherapy: getting to know the person properly and to understand exactly what they wanted in terms of change. Most psychiatrists do not have a first interview lasting four hours—someone with severe personality disorder deserves that time.

This interview was very important in setting the tasks ahead. It was clear that she had very serious traumatic experiences that would have to be addressed at some point. It was also obvious that, at present, she was so emotionally unstable that it was difficult to move forward in any direction. Although she had a serious personality disorder linked to this, it was complicated by a significant degree of pathological depression, social anxiety, and panic, symptoms that she unfortunately dealt with frequently by drinking. This was a combined mental state and personality problem, a true Galenic syndrome.

It was not being treated well. Unfortunately, like many people who are given a diagnosis of emotionally unstable personality disorder, she was being treated with six different drugs, some of which had led to dependence and others that seemed to have absolutely no efficacy. I made it clear that some of these drugs would have to be withdrawn, but this would be done with her agreement at an appropriate time. She agreed to this.

Although her past trauma was such an important part of her pathology, it could not be dealt with adequately at this time. The most important aspect of this was the need to change her life course. I sometimes give advice here in 21 words—'I am what I am, I am what I have been, what I will be is not what I have been'. In the longer term, we had to change Melanie's life plans drastically.

What bothered Melanie most was the implication that, whatever she did, she would always be rejected for any substantial treatment because, as the trust put it, she was 'too vulnerable'. I will leave it to the reader to decide exactly what is meant by this statement. I think it means 'too difficult to handle'. The notion that she could not have a care coordinator because she would become over-dependent on a person was something I had never come across before. Dependence should not be treated by rejection.

When I made my first assessment, Melanie was managing her dependence in a very unsatisfactory way. She had a paid carer, who was also depressed and unhappy and who tended to drink to excess. The relationship was not helping either of them, but Melanie was afraid to let it go.

Reluctantly, I had to accept that, at present in particular, Melanie was very highly dependent, and this would not change quickly. We had to both acknowledge this and use it constructively. If Melanie's dependence could be transferred to me and shared with another, this could offer a way forward. So I needed to stress, first of all, that I would retain regular contact with her for six months at least but linked this with a promise to me that she would make no suicide attempts or self-harm episodes of any kind in the next six months. Most people would claim this to be a very rash requirement for someone who had been harming themselves so frequently. But it turned out to be a positive transaction. I explained this by emphasising that if she repeatedly self-harmed and was admitted to hospitals in different parts of the country, this continuity of care would disappear, and therapy and any other form of treatment would be compromised. Because I also recognised that the problem of changing staff in her previous care was a major fear, I confirm that I would continue to see her over the six-month period if she avoided self-harm. What the trust regarded as a major reason for not giving her a care coordinator, the presence of excessive dependence, was used as a positive by me. By confirming that I would not reject her care if she helped me in this respect, I recognise that I was fostering dependence in some way, but I was using it as a lever to establish a therapeutic relationship.

She agreed to this requirement also, and, surprisingly, she followed through for the six-month period. (But read later about what happened subsequently.) I also discussed with her the long-term goals that she wanted to achieve. Although many might consider this type of discussion inappropriate at a time of crisis, I wanted to set the nidotherapy boundaries at an early stage. She said she wanted to leave the house where she had been born, abused, and damaged throughout her life, and she also wanted to overcome the many traumatic experiences she had been through from the age of three onward.

It can be seen immediately that this type of problem cannot be addressed easily by a formal diagnosis. If you wanted to make one in Melanie's case, it would be severe personality disorder with strong representation from the negative affective and impulsive domains, together with generalised anxiety, social anxiety disorder, panic, moderately severe depression, complex post-traumatic stress disorder (Karatzias et al., 2023) and harmful alcohol use. In the near future, there is likely to be a change in the funding of mental health services. This will involve a change from funding through activity (i.e., number of patients seen and time spent in community and inpatient settings) to one based on diagnosis. Personality disorder is one of the important groups of diagnosis, but all the other diagnoses would be taken into account in determining the costs of care that would be planned. The personality disorder would be the diagnosis with the highest cost implications, but the others would all contribute as well.

Stage 2 in nidotherapy—environmental analysis

It was established very early on in my assessment that the environment in which Melanie had lived for almost every year since her birth was a toxic one. Even in her adolescence and as a young woman, she had been gang raped close to where she lived. So the house where she lived and all the immediate streets were surrounded by full of memories of childhood abuse. This could not be a place which could be included as part of her therapy.

But it was not possible to change her accommodation immediately. Because her needs were so pronounced, it would be necessary for her to have some form of institutional care. Inpatient psychiatric care was the least desirable of these, not least because Melanie had so many bad experiences in the past. There are also specialist personality disorder services in many parts of the country, but the local service had been rejected by the trust and was not residential. One pathway which is being used increasingly more often for those with severe personality disorder (mainly emotional instability) in the United Kingdom is referral to a private hospital at a different location (often called out-of-area placements), where there are personality disorder services which are funded by the NHS if the referral comes from a mental health trust. These now are costing over £2M annually and account for more than one in five of all out-of-area placements (Mizen et al., 2025).

As these were not available at the time Reece and I, representing NIDUS-UK, took on her care, we had to think of other possibilities. Reece had a number of contacts with solicitors, NHS administrators, and local authority officials, and they provided him with valuable advice. This phase of nidotherapy is called environmental advocacy, and in Mel's case, we had to pursue advocacy with persistence and gusto as so many doors had already been closed. The phases of adaptation described in Chapter 5 under the acronym CALMED all had to employed at different times. There were confrontations with the mental health trust over their dereliction of care; avoidance of outright anger and criticism as it would have been counter-productive; leverage in the form of support from managers, and, in Melanie's case, her GP (who helped greatly in medication reduction); modifications to our strategy for the right institutional care when initial plans went awry; escape into a brief holiday when Melanie and her family went to Corfu; and dissociation, the last component of CALMED, when Melanie decided that the only way forward was to change her name to Tyrer and have a completely new identity.

By the end of this period, December 2023, we had completed an environmental plan. Its components were (a) her carer would be advised to leave, and as he had other accommodation, this was quite possible; (b) a new consultant had been identified within the trust who had generously taken on Melanie's consultant supervision, even though this was not in his job description, and he was doing a big favour by taking on this task; and (c) finding residential support for Melanie away from the family home was now a necessity as the first stage in managing her trauma.

Stage 3—finding a therapeutic community

With the agreement of the new consultant, referral was made to a nearby rehabilitation unit run as a therapeutic community. But when we visited and assessed the environment there, it was not too encouraging. Most of the residents were relatively uncommunicative, and many suffered from autistic spectrum disorder. Several had stayed there for many years, and this was a worry as Melanie was keen on moving forward much more quickly.

Despite these concerns, we felt we had to make the most of this possibility, and Melanie accepted the place that was offered there. Unfortunately, matters went wrong quickly. There were very few interactive sessions with other residents and staff, and Melanie became increasingly frustrated. She was then spat at and verbally assaulted by another resident and found this so disturbing she returned home before deciding to return to the unit. Although efforts were made to calm down the situation with appropriate apologies, these did not go anywhere, and eventually, the placement had to be abandoned.

There was then an unusual hiatus. Melanie said to a train driver that she was feeling suicidal and wanted to jump under a train. He placed her in his cabin and arranged for her transfer to hospital, where she was assessed and put under a section of the Mental Health Act. There were no beds available, so she was transferred to a personality disorder unit at a private hospital—now a standard procedure when there are insufficient beds available and no other placements are suitable.

One advantage of private hospitals is their living arrangements. They are much more pleasant places to stay then acute psychiatric wards in general hospitals, and there is no constant pressure to discharge back to the community. Paradoxically, it could be argued that there is a perverse incentive to discharge because the longer the patient states in hospital, the greater the income accruing to the private hospital. But the important factor in this admission was that Melanie was treated respectfully, had her problems listened to at length, and received valuable support from a psychologist. This gave her a degree of encouragement that was to prove useful at the next stage of care.

Stage 4—addressing depression and the traumatic past

Melanie continued to have predictable traumatic memories from her past when she returned home. She also became more severely depressed, and her consultant approved a course of modified electroconvulsive therapy (ECT). After six treatments for depression, she had improved significantly, but this made her even more determined to find a placement where her traumatic past could be addressed.

Melanie herself looked up these possibilities on the internet, and one that seemed most suitable was explored fully. Discussions took place with other psychiatrists who had referred patients there with positive results; it was felt that this was the most likely type of accommodation to address Melanie's many emotional needs. A strong case for referral to the one that seemed most suitable (Khiron) was made, and this was presented to the referral panel. These panels have great difficulty in deciding which of these applications (called extra-contractual referrals) should be approved and which not.

At the point of writing, we do not know if Melanie will be funded to attend the therapeutic community. But we are confident it will happen at some point. Where nidotherapy has been of help at various points in this saga is, in her words, 'It has given me hope to know that some have faith in me and have not rejected me from help like so many others'.

Nidotherapy has maintained continuity through all the ups and downs and geographical movements, has harnessed many advocates and supporters along the way, has listened carefully to what she wants and acted in her wishes, and has kept the main environmental need—the move to a different setting from the house where she grew up and was abused—in constant focus. It has a clear pathway and a definite ending.

I end this chapter with a comment about selfishness. Selfishness is a personality trait particularly associated with psychopathy and antisocial behaviour that has little social value and is generally discouraged. But sufferers of all mental illnesses have the tendency to selfishness, the concern about their own troubles that seems to suppress any concern they have over other people's feelings and reactions. This is quite normal; you are bound to give selective attention to your own troubles when they dominate your consciousness and squeeze out the normal concerns you have for others. The idea that those with personality disorder should be dealt with at arm's length because they will exploit and manipulate your emotions so you become a slave to their demands is utterly wrong. We all have the capacity to take advantage of the goodwill of others; it goes with the territory of care. It is not a reason to relinquish continuing help for those who are on a complicated rocky road to recovery.

References

Bach B, Simonsen E, Kongerslev MT, Bo S, Hastrup LH, Simonsen S, et al. (2023). ICD-11 personality disorder features in the Danish general population: cut-offs and prevalence rates for severity levels. *Psychiatry Research*, 328, 115484.

Karatzias T, Bohus M, Shevlin M, Hyland P, Bisson JI, Roberts N, et al. (2023). Distinguishing between ICD-11 complex post-traumatic stress disorder and borderline personality disorder: clinical guide and recommendations for future research. *British Journal of Psychiatry*, 223, 403–406.

Mizen S, Jones V, & Howson S (2025). Out of area placements for people with "personality disorder": making the case for a local intensive psychotherapeutic alternative. *Personality and Mental Health*, 19, e1649.

Neves Horácio A, Bento A, & Gama Marques J (2023). Personality and attachment in the homeless: a systematic review. *International Journal of Social Psychiatry*, 69, 1312–1326.

World Health Organisation (2024). *Clinical Descriptions and Diagnostic Requirements for ICD-11 Mental, Behavioural and Neurodevelopmental Disorders.* WHO: Geneva.

Yang M, Coid J, & Tyrer P (2010). A national survey of personality pathology recorded by severity. *British Journal of Psychiatry*, 197, 193–199.

Chapter 19

Personality disorder and stigma

Discrimination against people with mental illness is getting less but is still very strong. In a wide-ranging treatise on the subject, Graham Thornicroft summarises its features:

> [D]iscrimination against the mentally ill is still a major problem throughout the world. It can manifest itself in subtle ways, such as the terminology used to describe the person or their illness, or in more obvious ways—by the way the mentally ill might be treated and deprived of basic human rights. Should we just accept such discrimination as deeply rooted and resistant to change, or is this something that we can collectively change if we understand and commit ourselves to tackling the problem?
>
> (Thornicroft, 2020)

Thornicroft shows that we, as providers of mental health services, together with those who receive them, can act to reduce this discrimination, and he gives many examples of this in his book. But how should we go about it? There are two types of campaigners against stigma: the avoiders and the acceptors. The avoiders argue that either the subject giving rise to stigma does not exist and needs to be refashioned, or, if it does exist, it should never be mentioned. The acceptors argue the opposite viewpoint. They feel the subject does exist but has been misrepresented and needs to be exposed in its proper light. The avoiders promote stigma; the acceptors reduce it.

Many years ago, we came across an example of both these groups. I was one of six callow youths on a university expedition to central Africa, and our initial base was in Johannesburg where we hired all our transport and materials. We had dinner with a close family friend when we arrived. He was a liberal campaigner before he left England, and he seemed to be similar when we met him in Johannesburg. But when we brought up the subject of race, he did not want to talk about it. He insisted that he was against

DOI: 10.4324/9781003560630-19

racism but gave no examples of this even though they were all around him. He worked for an insurance company, drove into work every day, and had very little contact with any black people apart from those working in his office. We had no real conversation about racism because, in his mind, it had been excluded as too sensitive a subject.

This was very different from our own experience. Because we made way for people of all races when we were walking round the main streets of Johannesburg, within a few minutes, we were invited into a banned meeting of the African National Congress and given a basic lesson about the evils of apartheid. 'Remember this when you go back home to England', we were told.

Stigma about personality disorder unfortunately has more supporters for the avoider approach than that the acceptor one. It has come to be regarded in the same way as racism, with any mention of the subject labelled rapidly as an example of stigma. So nowadays, any mention of a racial term, almost in any context, is regarded as racist (McWhorter, 2021). Loose language has become toxic. I have illustrated this in a cat satire in which cats with large ears (macropinnates) have dominated cats with small ears (macropinnates) for generations, and a campaign to remove 'pinnarism', as it is called, has become so intense that the word 'ear' has been removed from vocabulary. The consequences are far from pleasant (Tyrer, 2023).

An example of how the avoider approach leads to greater stigma and damage comes from a recent experience at the Royal College of Psychiatrists. A distinguished researcher in forensic psychiatry was asked some years ago to host a seminar for colleagues on personality disorder. These seminars were held annually and were always heavily oversubscribed. In advertising the latest of these two years ago, he referred to some of the people with antisocial features as being like 'a thorn in the flesh'. This was immediately picked up on by an expert by experience working with the college and an immediate complaint made to the president of the college. He responded by issuing a public apology on the college website, cancelling the seminar, and stating that it would be replaced by a teaching programme that was more acceptable.

The seminar was duly cancelled and never replaced, and now this teaching programme is no more. What has been gained by this? Has it reduced stigma? No, it has accentuated the language of stigma unnecessarily, led to a reduction in teaching and understanding, and sent out a warning to others that any negative comments about those with personality problems is likely to be dealt with by a severe response from the Royal College. This will inhibit researchers from doing research in the area in the same way in which anger from many has inhibited research into chronic fatigue syndrome. Is this really the way we want to be going in understanding personality disorder and reducing stigma: making it an ocean of stigma and a desert of knowledge?

When people criticise psychiatrists who work in the field of personality disorder and claim they are promoting stigma, I do hope they realise they are not the only ones who suffer. The cat in Disney's *Cinderella* is not like Jessica Rabbit. He's not just drawn bad; he is bad. He is called Lucifer, and he is scheming and wicked, shouting 'I am an antisocial personality disorder' every time he appears. Psychiatrists working with those who have personality disorder are portrayed as Lucifer equivalents, and their motivation is always to create conflict and harm.

In the last two years, there has been a thorough review of the subject of personality disorder from an expert reference group that has been highly concerned about prejudice and discrimination in the subject. I have been a member of the group but have not had much success in promoting the message of Chapter 2 in this book: that the ICD-11 classification of personality disorder should have a major effect on reducing stigma because the dimension of personality disturbance includes almost everybody in the population.

After the end of this exercise, six principles have now been generated about the diagnosis of personality disorder. These may not be the final ones, and I have made my concerns known to the group. In each of them, we see all the evidence of avoidance of the diagnosis rather than acceptance, and so I view the publication of these recommendations with foreboding.

Here are the six principles and my comments in response.

Principle 1. We need to start with an acknowledgment of harm the particular wording used in the label/diagnosis does to many people, as a result of both the response, attitudes and culture it evokes from services and the clinicians and professionals in them. For many it is seen/used as tantamount to an insult and therefore it can negatively impact an individual's sense of self and self-esteem. This includes but is not limited to the specific term 'personality disorder'. It can also lead to the denial of certain treatments or a belief that certain approaches won't work. This is particularly so where children and young people are concerned, when told at a young age that they could have a personality that is disordered. This is a sense that is shared by many clinicians too who are taught and work in a system that created this and that they would rather move away from.

There are two components to this recommendation: the statement that the words 'personality disorder' create harm and are 'tantamount to insult' and the implication that the condition is untreatable. Both of them come into the avoider stigma strategy. This is expressed in its most severe form by those who say that even the mention of the words 'personality disorder' is so damaging it is retraumatising. (The same reaction is created by 'ear' in my book—Tyrer, 2023.) To understand why these two words are considered so damaging, it is worth reminding ourselves of the settings in which the diagnosis of personality disorder is mentioned. Perhaps the most frequent is the accident and emergency department of a general hospital when a patient is seen following an episode of self harm. The staff who use the words 'personality disorder' in a dismissive way in this setting are usually general nurses who have no particular knowledge of psychiatry, are often overworked and under stress, and are irritated by people who have not been harmed by events beyond their control but have harmed themselves deliberately.

The use of the term 'personality disorder' as a loose throwaway in this context is unforgivable, but it is not the diagnosis that is at fault; it is the person who uses it who should be taken aside and trained in mental health literacy.

The second implication that the condition is untreatable is plainly wrong, and if no other message manages to emanate from this book, the one I would choose above all others is that personality disorder is not permanent. The impression that the condition is untreatable is reinforced by clinical teams who refuse to take patients into their care if the words 'emotional instability' are mentioned in the referral documents. The reaction in these settings runs along the lines of 'We want easy patients who are going to work well together and not cause any trouble with our special treatments. Those with emotional instability are well known for causing trouble and conflict, so we must exclude them'. There is also a high degree of ignorance in this set of beliefs that needs to be corrected by training. This undoubtedly indicates discrimination, but suggesting that 'clinicians too who are taught and work in a system that created this and that they would rather move away from' is not a correct description. The clinicians (including nurses and support workers) who are preventing the access of patients in this way are not following a broken diagnostic system; they are simply exploiting prejudice. It would help enormously if we could properly classify emotional dysregulation in a way that gave it more meaning, but at present, every half-trained mental health worker can parrot 'borderline' with eye-rolling to their friends and giggle behind their cupped hands with impunity because this word has lost all meaning. Personality disorder should not be stained by association with it.

Principle 2. Our recommendation is therefore to move towards a new system of classification that seeks to validate rather than stigmatise—one that describes the context, rather than labelling the individual. We would like to advocate for a reconceptualisation that moves the focus from deficit to response to one's environment and from an exclusive focus on the individual to a focus on the experiences and relationships around them. These are recommendations we make to those engaged in the update of systems of classification like ICD and DSM.

It is very difficult to make sense of this particular recommendation. As far as I know, no diagnosis in psychiatry is made as a 'deficit to response in one's environment' unless this is an oblique reference to post-traumatic stress disorder. Similarly, there is no diagnosis that focuses on experiences and relationships except by saying that, in personality disorders, these tend to be disturbed. In asking for an update to ICD and DSM, it is to be noted that ICD-11 has only just been published 30 years after ICD-10 and is unlikely to be altered within the next few decades, and DSM has had a few bruising encounters after revising its wording too rapidly in previous years, and it may take some time before DSM-6 appears.

The decision to formalise a diagnosis is a complex one. It can be improved, and people with lived experience should have more say in what is decided, but it is governed by many influences. Personality disorder was first classified by the French psychiatrist Philippe Pinel in 1801 as 'emotional insanity', described as 'a sort of instinctual fury, as though only the affective faculties had been impaired' (Shorter, 2005, p. 213), a pretty good description of emotional dysregulation that has lasted over 200 years, so the terms are not likely to be abandoned without very good reason. Hours of work with psychiatrists across the world go into revisions of diagnoses, and great efforts have to be made to get agreement. The early international efforts all failed because of opposition, mainly from psychoanalysts, and the final agreements are hard won. The impression they are given casually without evidence is completely wrong.

> Principle 3. The way the diagnosis is reached needs to be fundamentally changed. It is often a reflexive response from clinicians and, consciously or not, used in a pejorative way as an emotional reaction. Acknowledging the propensity for this is a starting point and this needs to be replaced with more a relational culture that is more collaborative and less hierarchical. Training around new ways of working is therefore crucial so that every interaction with any health or care professional has the potential to be a therapeutic and collaborative sense-making one.

If a diagnosis is made as an emotional reaction to a situation, it is clearly an error, and nobody would disagree with this. Unfortunately we have moved from the position in the past when psychiatric diagnosis was just shared between professionals as a means of rapid communication—in effect, a form of shorthand to pass on information economically—to the present day, when every person seems to have awareness of the subject of diagnosis and feels it is perfectly reasonable to change it in light of their own experiences. In the case of problems arising from personality, it is perfectly fair to say that a collective description is inadequate because every personality is unique, but it is quite another matter to say they cannot be classified at all. Those who support the Power Threat Meaning Framework want to abandon all 'medical' words like 'symptoms', 'disorder', and 'diagnosis' and replace them with a different system that acknowledges that social and interpersonal factors are often the cause of distress and need to be included in the diagnostic system (Boyle & Johnstone, 2020). Yes, of course, symptoms and distress need to be acknowledged in every therapeutic encounter, but you cannot create a classification system based on these alone. You have to join up common features in every classification. It can't be done by 'training in new ways of working'; that is not a framework for any form of systematic enquiry. A good classification has to have clinical utility; it must make sense and be helpful to a large number of practitioners applying many different forms of treatment. Creating one from the stories of distressed patients cannot have this commonality; each is a story that stands on its own but cannot be combined into a useful grouping. If we abandoned diagnosis in psychiatry, we would return to the dark ages in which every therapeutic encounter would be an exercise in guesswork. We would not be able to make use of previous knowledge except by comparing our own experience with past patients who have been seen. A good diagnosis conveys basic information to both health professional and patient, and this has to be in a form that is understood clearly by both. It is the last part of this exercise that is most important in getting rid of stigma.

> Principle 4. It needs to be emphasised that many people have other diagnoses, which often need to be considered first and as an alternative, where appropriate. Most commonly these include PTSD, PMDD, neurodivergence and bipolar affective disorder. These are categories that are often considered to be more helpful and less harmful as a way of understanding one's experience.

This is a very dangerous suggestion. It implies that all the difficulties that are present in people with personality disorder can be explained by other terms which are less stigmatising and therefore could be used instead. But just consider how this would work in practice. A person who has mood swings as part of their personality disorder is seen and re-diagnosed as having bipolar disorder. The main treatments for bipolar disorder are psychopharmacological, and they have an excellent evidence base. But there is no evidence that those with personality disorder respond to the drugs that are effective in bipolar disorder (National Institute for Health and Care Excellence, 2009; Stoffers-Winterling et al., 2022), so re-diagnosing would be a pathway to unnecessary polypharmacy.

The other implication of this recommendation is that no form of management of the personality disorder is effective, whereas those for neurodivergence and complex post-traumatic stress disorder are much more likely to lead to recovery. This is not true. It could be argued that these diagnostic terms are more acceptable than personality disorder, but it does not alter the fact that they are very difficult to manage, and there are no clear evidence-based treatments.

> Principle 5. A fundamental foundation of a new approach to diagnosing and diagnosis, needs to be the utilisation of comprehensive psychological formulation as a core aspect of the way people are connected to, understood and understand themselves, within the framework of a wider bio-psycho-social approach.

This is the most reasonable principle of the six that have been formulated. All psychiatrists are trained to complete their assessment of a patient using a detailed formulation (Owen et al., 2014), and this is an important accompaniment that does not replace a diagnosis but adds flesh to it. It is also relevant that a bald diagnosis of personality disorder given to a patient is not going to be greeted with the same degree of acceptance as one of depressive disorder. In our own practice we often introduce the subject in these words:

> [A]t present your personality function is poor, and that it is contributing to your distress. We must take this into account when deciding how to help you. This does not mean that you necessarily have a personality disorder as this could easily change.
>
> (Tyrer & Mulder, 2022, p. 12)

> Principle 6. The diagnosis needs to be arrived at in a more collaborative way, with more equality between the clinician and the patient in determining it. It also needs to be more dynamic in that it should be understood as something that is subject to change over time and therefore clinicians should be open to regularly reviewing it and, again, this also needs to be done in a relational, collaborative and less hierarchical way.

This recommendation also contains a great deal of sense. One of the most damaging features of the diagnosis of personality disorder is the implication of permanence. By saying to people that they may be temporarily showing all the features of personality disorder and, if necessary, pointing these out in detail, one of the first steps of understanding can be achieved. I once gave a lecture on personality disorder to a large audience of professionals and people who had been diagnosed with personality disorder and made a joke about drama queens. I was heavily criticised by the audience at question time and subsequently at the end of the meeting, and it was pointed out to me, quite correctly, that I was showing evidence of my impulsive and somewhat exhibitionistic personality in making this joke and creating upset in others. When I enquired further, I was told that this was not the first time I had shown this behaviour, and so I should think further about correcting it. I was actually attracting attention in the wrong sort of way. I hope this gave me a degree of insight into my personality and helped me prevent making the same mistake in future.

I am not suggesting that someone with more severe personality disturbance would immediately take corrective action in the same way that I have tried to do, but by giving feedback about behaviour, you are giving much more valuable information than a simple diagnostic term.

A positive message of acceptance of personality disorder

If I was given a free hand in composing advice to reduce stigma in the acceptor rather than the avoider form, it would have these five components.

1.   We are all on a spectrum of personality disturbance

Our personalities are created by a mix of our inherited genes and our life experience. At various times in our lives, our personalities may lead to problems, so we become disturbed. These can be corrected by making adjustments so we can move along the spectrum to a better position.

2.   Personality disturbance is not permanent

Although our basic personalities do not change much, at times they can lead to more disturbance than others. All such disturbance can be temporary if the right corrective action is taken.

3.   There is nothing wrong in accepting you have a personality problem

As we all have some degree of personality disturbance, we need to come to terms with it and, if we are brave, share it with others. This will help people understand us better. Do not be afraid to ask your therapists, 'What do you think of my personality? Are there problems that might need to be addressed?' It will help them to respond if you initiate this.

4. *People with different personalities should be allowed, if they so wish, to celebrate their differences, not forced to change unless they have dissocial tendencies that need attention to protect society*

We do not live in a society where everyone is the same. This would be a very boring place. Some are very different from the people we expect to see, but that makes them more interesting. Oddness adds spice to life.

5. *There are many ways of helping people get over personality problems; they do not last*

If I have only succeeded in getting over one message in this book, I hope it is that personality problems change over time. When people claim their lives have been permanently damaged by their genes, their early environmental trauma, and the interactions between them, they are wrong. Damage to personality is not destruction. All those who doubt this should read Joel Paris's book *Myths of Trauma: Why Adversity Does Not Necessarily Make Us Sick* (Paris, 2022). The mix of intelligence, personality strengths, the neuroplasticity of the brain, and the environment in all its forms represents powerful restitution; we just need to harness these assets and not despair.

6. *Do not allow self-stigma to take over*

One of the by-products of campaigns against stigma is that they draw attention to conditions that may be dormant but are then highlighted into consciousness. This can be viewed positively and lead to change for the better but can also have a negative effect, particularly marked in those who have the conditions that have received greater exposure (Smith, 2013). When this extends to those with a borderline diagnosis having their symptoms of life-threatening physical illness ignored (Navarre, 2025), we have a serious problem on our hands. The possession of this diagnosis leads to greater self-stigma. As one of my patients said to me, 'Ten years ago, I wanted my diagnosis changed to borderline personality disorder so I could have treatment. Now I wish I had never received this diagnosis; I'm ashamed to admit it, and I want it taken away from my records'.

One of the main advantages of the ICD-11 dimensional system is that there is no reason for either stigma or self-stigma. When King Edward VII said in 1909, 'We are all socialists now', he surprised many. But at that time, everyone was supporting the budget reforms of David Lloyd George, which brought everyone into the socialist fold. The same applies to personality disorder; we all need to champion it as owners of the condition. 'We are all personality disordered now', I can hear King Charles say, and he has the knowledge and understanding of the subject to make this possible. He wrote in 1993, '[T]he challenge to mental health can never be addressed without all involved in health care working together to empower every potential patient, as far as can be, to care for their own mental health' (HRH Prince of Wales, 1993).

The celebration of personality difficulties should never cease. We need to promote their assets at least as much as their problems, and if we had exercised this more actively in the past, the suffering of Ludwig van Beethoven, Vincent van Gogh, Howard Hughes, Melanie Lukeman, and Jessica Rabbit would have been replaced by praise and commendation for their honesty and bravery.

References

Boyle H & Johnstone L (2020). *A Straight Talking Introduction to the Power Threat Meaning Framework: An Alternative to Psychiatric Diagnosis.* PCCS Books.

HRH Prince of Wales (1993). Foreword. In: P Tyrer, R Higgs, & G Strathdee (eds.), *Mental Health and Primary Care: A Changing Agenda.* Gaskell Books, Royal College of Psychiatrists.

McWhorter J (2021). *Woke Racism: How a New Religion Has Betrayed Black America.* Forum.

National Institute for Health and Care Excellence (2009). *Borderline Personality Disorder: Recognition and Management* (NICE Clinical Guideline CG78). London: NICE.

Navarre KM (2025). "You sure she's not making this up?": a qualitative investigation of stigma toward adults with borderline personality disorder in physical healthcare settings. *Personality and Mental Health*, 19, e1646.

Owen G, Wessely S, & Murray R (2014). *The Maudsley Handbook of Practical Psychiatry* (6th edition). Oxford Medical Publications.

Paris J (2022). *Myths of Trauma: Why Adversity Does Not Necessarily Make Us Sick.* Oxford University Press.

Shorter E (2005). *A Historical Dictionary of Psychiatry.* Oxford University Press.

Smith M (2013). Anti-stigma campaigns: time to change. *British Journal of Psychiatry*, 202, s49–s50.

Stoffers-Winterling JM, Storebø OJ, Pereira Ribeiro J, Kongerslev MT, Völlm BA, Mattivi JT, et al. (2022). Pharmacological treatment for borderline personality disorder. *Cochrane Database of Systematic Reviews*, 1114, CD012956.

Tyrer P (2023). *The Pinnarism Project.* Lincoln: Impspired.

Tyrer P & Mulder R (2022). *Personality Disorder: From Evidence to Understanding.* Cambridge University Press.

Glossary

As much as possible, the technical terms described in this book have been defined and developed in language that is easily understood. This glossary aims to provide a background to some of the terminology that requires additional description.

Acceptance and commitment therapy: This is a form of psychotherapy that does not aim to remove unpleasant symptoms but asks the sufferer to accept and come to terms with them instead of being in a constant battle. It adds a focus on commitment to actions that are linked to long-term, healthy, and constructive goals.

Addiction: The inability to stop any activity or behaviour because of its perceived reward that is so strong it ignores negative consequences.

ADHD: Attention deficit-hyperactivity disorder (ADHD) is characterised by three elements: inability to concentrate because of inattention (attention deficit), overly active behaviour (hyperactivity), poor concentration and distractibility, usually summarised as impulsivity. It is a condition that has been diagnosed much more often in recent years, particularly in children, with some saying that one in five children are affected. This almost certainly is too high. Many feel the increase has been fanned by social media.

Anankastia: This is the new noun for obsessionality in ICD-11. To avoid confusion with obsessive-compulsive disorder, the ICD system has always coded the obsessional personality as anankastic personality. It arises from the Greek word *anankastikos,* meaning compulsion.

Asperger's syndrome: Asperger's syndrome is a condition first described by Hans Asperger but developed as a new disorder by Lorna Wing. It is best described as a mild variant of autistic spectrum disorder. It is not in the ICD-11 classification system.

Autistic spectrum disorder: A spectrum of conditions (like that of personality disorder) which extends from mild detachment and preference for few relationships to a severe disorder, often associated with intellectual disability, in which there is severe disability in communication, rigidity of behaviour and great difficulty in processing information. There is some overlap with personality disorder.

Autonomy: The ability to make decisions independently without external control. One of the aims of nidotherapy is to promote autonomy and so improve life satisfaction.

Bipolar disorder (formerly manic-depressive psychosis): A serious psychiatric disorder in which moods change from severe depression and hopelessness to excessive self-confidence and elevated mood (hypomania or mania depending on severity). In general, the depressive episodes in bipolar disorder are more common than the manic episodes. The main treatment for bipolar disorder is drugs, although some benefit has been shared with cognitive behaviour therapy and family-orientated approaches. In the ICD-11 classification, bipolar II disorder has also been introduced. There is a danger that this can be confused with the emotional instability of borderline personality problems and inappropriate treatment with drugs given if true bipolar disorder is not present.

Borderline: This is an unhappy adjective that has been wrongly attached to personality disorder and has created nothing but confusion. In some ways, it is an accurate adjective. It does not belong anywhere; it only skulks on the borders between personality, emotions, mental illness, and normal function. Because it is such an elastic adjective, it can be applied to almost any negative interaction between people. It is a term that has lost all meaning and will soon be relegated to the history books.

Classification: Any system that organises a set of information into groups.

Cognitive behaviour therapy: A psychotherapy that attempts to alter inappropriate emotions, thoughts, and behaviours by challenging irrational beliefs. It is most commonly used with common mental disorders but has been extended to personality disorders.

Complex post-traumatic stress disorder: A more complicated form of post-traumatic stress disorder in which the time between the stress and exhibition of the disorder can be delayed, often for many years. There are many who have suffered trauma in early years and develop personality problems in adult life. When these are clearly linked to the traumatic experiences, it is right to make this diagnosis.

Cost effectiveness: The measure of value for money. In mental health, a highly cost-effective intervention is one which costs little and leads to great gain. An intervention could also be regarded as cost effective if it creates more value at the same cost as a standard treatment. Nidotherapy has been one of the few psychological interventions that have been shown to be both very cheap and yet has created considerable gain.

Dependence: An abnormal degree of reliance, on another person, object, or activity.

Dialectical behaviour therapy: The best known of all psychological treatments for personality disorder introduced by Marsha Linehan. It particularly focuses on strategies and skills for dealing with emotional dysregulation and is, consequently, highly effective. But it is of limited value in most personality disorders if emotional instability is not present.

Dissociation: A mental state in which a person becomes detached from reality. In mild form, this can consist of only depersonalisation (feeling unreal) or derealisation (the surroundings feeling unreal), but in more severe cases, the person loses contact with their identity and cannot relate. An extreme form of dissociation is dissociative identity disorder (DID), in which the person changes personality dramatically and behaves in a completely different way from their normal state. This was first described by Robert Louis Stevenson in his book The *Strange Case of Dr Jekyll and Mr Hyde.*

Hoarding disorder: A condition, often linked to anankastic personality disorder, in which the sufferer finds it difficult to discard possessions that are of no further use, the consequence of which is excessive cluttering of objects that completely fill the person's property and greatly disrupt normal living. There is persistent difficulty discarding possessions, leading to excessive accumulation and domestic chaos that disrupt daily life.

International Classification of Diseases: The classification of all diseases, both physical and mental, first introduced in 1900 and regularly revised ever since. ICD-11 is the latest revision and was formally introduced in January 2022. The revisions are made over a period of many years with contributors from all parts of the world. It is necessary to ensure that all countries adopt the classification system so there is a common language across culture and nations.

Mental health act: Every mental health act is a form of coercion to protect the public and ensure compliance with treatment, with the intention of promoting improvement through evidence-based treatments. Unfortunately, despite greater tolerance of mental health in the community the use of mental health acts as a form of coercion is not diminishing.

Mentalisation-based treatment (MBT):   MBT is a psychodynamically derived form of psychotherapy that aims to improve a person's capacity to mentalise, a word that describes the ability to understand and interpret their thoughts and feelings and those of others. It was developed by Anthony Bateman and Peter Fonagy and first used in the treatment of borderline personality disorder but has since been expanded to other forms of personality disorder, addiction and eating disorders.

Nidotherapy: Nidotherapy originates from the notion of the nest, or *nidus* (Latin). A bird's nest, or indeed any form of nest, is an environmental structure that accommodates any shape placed within it. The aim of nidotherapy is to help people to find the nest that most suits them in life. It is not a formal treatment but a set of guiding principles that enable people to change their environments to make a more suitable fit.

Personality: There are many accounts of personality in this book, but it still remains very difficult to define. It comprises all aspects of the ways in which a person reacts to others through their unique characteristics and behaviour. These include the way they normally adjust to others through their preferred inclinations (traits and domains), activities and interests, social functioning, goals and drives, self-awareness and identity, and emotional adjustment. It is influenced equally by genetic and environmental factors; the first of these is relatively fixed, but the second is much more fluid and can also interact with the genetic components (epigenetics). Although personality is often said to be a permanent, unchanging attribute, this is not strictly true (and is contradicted many times in this book). Personality is not the same as a fingerprint; it alters when it alteration finds and is a dynamic force that is always on the move.

Randomised controlled trial: A randomised controlled trial (RCT) is still considered to be the best way of determining the effectiveness of a treatment. It involves randomly assigning participants to either an experimental group or a control group to measure the effectiveness of any intervention. Although randomised controlled trials can be relatively easy in testing some treatments such as drugs, as the control treatment can be a dummy tablet (placebo), it is much more difficult with psychological treatments. This is because it is very difficult to get a suitable control treatment for a complex psychological issue (especially personality disorders) as the ideal control should be exactly the same as the experimental treatment in terms of its length and content with only the experimental treatment lacking. It is extremely difficult to get such a control for the complex treatment programmes necessary with personality disorder.

Royal College of Psychiatrists: This is the main professional organisation for psychiatrists in the United Kingdom. Similar national bodies include the American Psychiatric Association and the Royal Australian and New Zealand College of Psychiatrists. Note that psychologists have a separate body, the British Psychological Society, to represent them. The College is responsible as the official mouthpiece to represent psychiatrists, to promote psychiatric research, providing public information about mental health problems, and giving advice to those responsible for training and certifying psychiatrists in the UK.

Social prescribing: Social prescribing is an ill-defined term to describe the provision of a range of activities that are non-medical but focused on improving social and environmental change. It therefore overlaps with nidotherapy but has a more diffuse remit. In the UK it is mainly provided by link workers with good local knowledge who can advise on volunteering, artistic events and activities, group learning, gardening, befriending, cookery, healthy eating advice and a range of sports, all chosen with the intention of improving mental health.

Stigma: A word originally described as a lesion created on the skin of slaves to indicate inferiority but now expanded to include a wide range of inappropriately held negative attitudes and beliefs. These in the case of personality disorder include labelling (the automatic assumption of personal conflict), stereotyping (the belief that all are similarly afflicted), separation (exclusion and isolation of those individuals), and discrimination (unequal representation in society). Stigma can be shown by others or created by those affected, when it is known as self-stigma.

Trauma-informed therapy: This subject is becoming increasingly important in understanding the development of personality problems and how they should be managed. But it is difficult to establish the content of the therapy as opposed to its overarching principles. These principles include the creation of a trusting, safe, therapeutic environment, the encouragement of autonomy, respect for relevant cultural factors, understanding of the impact of trauma and a collaborative team approach. These help to create a trauma-conscious environment but do not in themselves constitute therapy. One key element seems to be disclosure; so many traumatic experiences are suppressed and hidden away, and once they have been brought to the surface it can be a great relief.

Index

For Product Safety Concerns and Information please contact our EU
representative GPSR@taylorandfrancis.com
Taylor & Francis Verlag GmbH, Kaufingerstraße 24, 80331 München, Germany

www.ingramcontent.com/pod-product-compliance
Lightning Source LLC
Chambersburg PA
CBHW070324270326
41926CB00017B/3743

9 781032 869513